www.wadsworth.com

wadsworth.com is the World Wide Web site for Wadsworth and is your direct source to dozens of online resources.

At *wadsworth.com* you can find out about supplements, demonstration software, and student resources. You can also send email to many of our authors and preview new publications and exciting new technologies.

wadsworth.com
Changing the way the world learns®

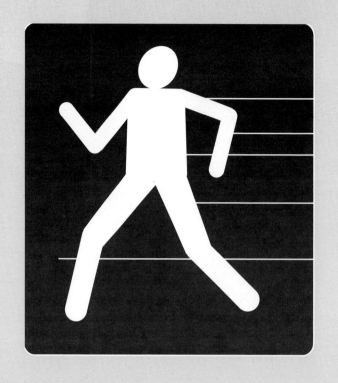

Walking & Jogging

For Health & Wellness

Fifth Edition

Frank Rosato

University of Memphis

THOMSON

WADSWORTH

Australia • Canada • Mexico • Singapore • Spain • United Kingdom • United States

THOMSON

™

WADSWORTH

Publisher: Peter Marshall
Acquisitions Editor: April Lemons
Assistant Editor: Andrea Kesterke
Technology Project Manager: Star MacKenzie
Marketing Manager: Jennifer Somerville
Marketing Assistant: Mona Weltmer
Advertising Project Manager: Shemika Britt
Project Manager, Editorial Production: Karen Haga

Print/Media Buyer: Barbara Britton
Permissions Editor: Elizabeth Zuber
Production Service and Compositor: Ash Street Typecrafters, Inc.
Text and Cover Designer: Harry Voigt
Copy Editor: Carolyn Acheson
Cover Images: Getty Images, Inc.
Text and Cover Printer: Transcontinental Printing, Inc.

Printed in Canada
4   5   6   7   06   05

For more information about our products, contact us at:
Thomson Learning Academic Resource Center
1-800-423-0563

For permission to use material from this text, contact us by:
Phone: 1-800-730-2214
Fax: 1-800-730-2215
Web: http://www.thomsonrights.com

Library of Congress Control Number: 2002108106

ISBN 0-534-51726-9

Wadsworth/Thomson Learning
10 Davis Drive
Belmont, CA 94002-3098
USA

Asia
Thomson Learning
5 Shenton Way #01-01
UIC Building
Singapore 068808

Australia
Nelson Thomson Learning
102 Dodds Street
South Melbourne, Victoria 3205
Australia

Canada
Nelson Thomson Learning
1120 Birchmount Road
Toronto, Ontario M1K 5G4
Canada

Europe/Middle East/Africa
Thomson Learning
High Holborn House
50/51 Bedford Row
London WC1R 4LR
United Kingdom

Latin America
Thomson Learning
Seneca, 53
Colonia Polanco
11560 Mexico D.F.
Mexico

Spain
Paraninfo Thomson Learning
Calle/Magallanes, 25
28015 Madrid, Spain

Contents

Preface

The fields of exercise science and health promotion are dynamic, and the pace of change is accelerating. What was considered to be an article of faith just 5 to 10 years ago may be discarded like a pair of worn-out walking or jogging shoes today. In this edition, new information has replaced outdated information, new trends have been identified, and the concepts and content of this book are supported primarily by research that has been reported since the fourth edition was published.

The focus of the fifth edition of *Walking and Jogging for Health and Wellness* is consistent with that of its predecessors: The emphasis remains on enhancing health and fitness. The objective is not to turn novice exercisers into fierce competitors, although the material in this edition and its intent does not preclude that outcome. But the primary purpose is to introduce novice exercisers to the benefits of walking and jogging, and to present persuasive and logical reasons why they should take the time and make the effort to include exercise in their daily lives. The emphasis is to encourage ordinary people to start moving to enhance their health, or to improve their physical appearance, or to develop physical fitness, or for other reasons.

This edition provides the guidelines for novices to begin and sustain a walking or jogging program safely and effectively. Also, veteran walkers and joggers may find information that is useful for motivation and for refining established programs.

This edition has been substantially revised, beginning with a change in the title of the book to *Walking and Jogging for Health and Wellness*. This reflects the progression from a lower-intensity, lower-impact mode of exercise to a higher-intensity, higher-impact mode. Of course, it is not necessary to progress from walking to jogging. This change would depend upon one's interests, needs, and goals. But information is provided for those who would like to move from one activity to the other.

The order of the chapters has been changed to better fit the specific needs of beginning exercisers. The former Chapter 3, "Guidelines for Walking and Jogging" has been split into Chapters 3 and 4. Chapter 3, now titled "Getting Started," has updated and expanded guidelines for exercise. This chapter includes information on exercise resources such as locating reliable and credible information for walkers and joggers, tips for selecting a personal trainer, and information on walking/running clubs, YMCAs, community fitness centers, health clubs, worksite wellness programs, and more. Chapter 4, entitled "Walking and Jogging for Health and Fitness," has been expanded by including the exercise needs of special populations such as the unique concerns of women—exercise during pregnancy, breast support particularly during high-impact activities—exercise for elderly people, the exercise needs of children and adolescents, and exercise for overweight and obese people.

"Prevention and Treatment of Walking and Jogging Injuries" has been moved from Chapter 8 to Chapter 5 so students will come in contact with this information before they get too deeply involved with their exercise program. As a result, the information contained in this chapter possibly will help to prevent an injury early in the program, or it may help the new exerciser recognize the signs and symptoms of an impending injury and how to apply the appropriate treatment. An addition to this discussion is iliotibial band injury, because it seems to be a common running injury. Other exercise concerns, such as the wisdom and efficacy of exercising during an illness and nutritional approaches for preventing and treating illnesses, have been added.

As exercise physiologists continuously refine terminology that more accurately reflects physiological processes, several new terms have been introduced in Chapter 6, "Physiological Adaptations of Walking and Jogging." New terms include *elevated post-exercise oxygen consumption* and *oxygen drift*. Several changes in the guidelines for fluid intake and replacement are discussed, and the concept of *hyponatremia* is introduced.

Chapter 7, "Nutrition for Active People," addresses the basics of nutrition. This chapter also covers the latest information on the effect of different types of dietary fats (good versus bad), the antioxidants, free radicals or oxidants, phytochemicals, phytoestrogens, phytomedicinals, and transfatty acids.

In the previous edition, Chapter 5 covered cardiovascular disease and other chronic diseases were covered in Chapter 6. In this new edition, those chapters are combined in a new, streamlined Chapter 8, "Reducing the Risk of Selected Diseases Through Exercise." The major risk factors for coronary heart disease have been identified as a result of newer research evidence, and these are included.

This edition is accompanied by an instructor's manual that should facilitate the preparation, delivery, and assessment of instructional and learning objectives. A sample class outline for a 15-week semester is suggested that provides the order of presentation for the material as well as a sense of pacing. Secondly, five to ten sample test questions have been developed from each of the chapters. And third, a final exam for the course is presented. The Instructor's Manual will be made available to qualified adopters. Please consult your local sales representative for details.

I would like to thank April Lemons, Editor for Health at Wadsworth, for many ideas that have contributed markedly to the revision of this text. Special thanks to Devonia Cage who, after putting in her regular day at work, took my handwritten manuscript home, where she quickly turned it into a computer-driven hard copy.

I also would like to thank the following reviewers for their time and comments: Joe Peeples, Costal Georgia Community College; and Stephanie Eaton Agosta, Ohio University, Lancaster.

Finally, I would like to thank my wife Pat for her patience and willingness to take on some of my home responsibilities while I was involved in this project.

Frank Rosato, Ed.D.
University of Memphis

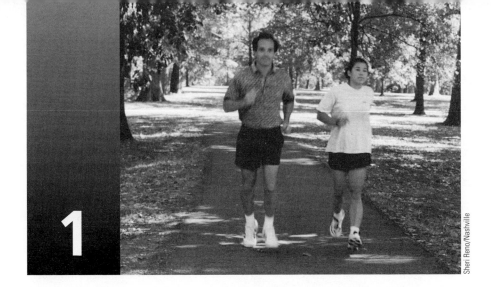

1

Physical Fitness: An Overview

Outline

National polls, surveys, and the mass media have documented the extent of the physical fitness movement in the United States. Further, studies regarding the cost-effectiveness of fitness and wellness programs in the workplace attests to their cost-effectiveness in terms of savings in health-care costs.

In this chapter you will be introduced to the extent of Americans' participation in exercise, its health benefits, and degrees of fitness. This chapter includes guidelines and rationales for exercise developed by the American College of Sports Medicine (ACSM) and the Centers for Disease Control and Prevention (CDC).

Some time-management tools are presented to help people find pockets of time during the day for worthwhile pursuits such as exercise. This chapter includes a rationale for choosing walking and jogging as safe and expeditious modes of activity for attaining physical fitness and enhancing health.

America on the Move

Throughout the United States we see people walking, jogging, cycling, and swimming to attain physical fitness,

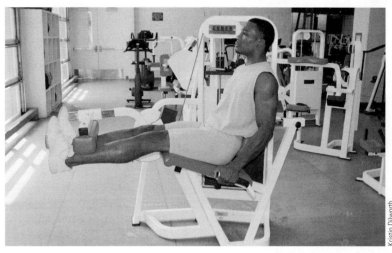

Kristin Dilworth

Exercise equipment is becoming more sophisticated.

weight loss, and other health-promoting benefits. Fitness clubs are packed with people doing aerobics to music and exercising with weights, stair-steppers, rowing machines, treadmills, and bikes. Exercise equipment is becoming more and more sophisticated every day. Information regarding fitness and health appears in the print and electronic media daily.

From this frenzy of activity, you easily could gain the perception that most Americans are fully involved in the exercise movement. Unfortunately, perception and reality are not the same. Information gathered during the last 30 years indicates that most Americans have not exercised enough to have a positive impact on their fitness level or their health status.

During the early years, literally millions of sedentary people began exercising aerobically and the movement grew rapidly. Eventually the influx of new participants slowed. In the past few years a disturbing trend has begun to surface: The exercise movement has reached a plateau in spite of growth in the population. This is occurring at a time when the health and wellness benefits associated with consistent participation in physical activities is most compelling.

Data accumulated on U. S. adults over the past couple of decades indicate that:[1]

1. Fifteen percent participate regularly (three times per week for at least 30 minutes) in vigorous physical activities that are not work-related

2. Twenty-two percent participate regularly (five times per week for at least 30 minutes) in sustained physical activity during nonworking hours

3. Twenty-five percent engage in no physical activity during nonworking hours

4. More than 60 percent engage in no exercise or participate sporadically or marginally, so no improvement in health status results

5. Only half of young people (12 to 21 years of age) participate regularly in vigorous physical activity

6. One-fourth of young people (12 to 21 years of age) report no participation at all.

A more recent survey by the International Health, Racquet, and Sports-club Association (IHRSA) adds further evidence to the contradiction that what Americans think about health enhancement and what they actually do to achieve it are essentially unrelated.[2] The top two priorities of the survey respondents were *maintaining good physical health* and *developing physical appearance*. The respondents rated these two factors higher than having more time for themselves, having good friends, having fulfilling relationships with their significant others, and reducing stress. The emphasis on physical appearance is surprising and ironic, considering that the Centers for Disease Control and Prevention announced findings in 2001 that a record 61 percent of American adults are overweight or obese.[3]

Answers by the survey respondents to several other questions indicated that they were unable to connect participation in exercise and the pursuit of physical fitness as primary vehicles to enhance their health and physical appearance. This may account for their unwillingness to put forth the effort to attain both of these goals.

Aerobic Exercise and Health

The trend toward exercise began in the 1960s with an emphasis on **aerobic exercise**, also referred to as **cardio-respiratory endurance** activities. The term *aerobic* literally means "with oxygen." When applied to exercise, it refers to lower intensity exercises of relatively long duration when the exerciser can supply the oxygen needed to meet the energy demands of the activity. Aerobic exercises are "steady state" or "pay as you go" exercises.

For the average healthy person, aerobic endurance can be improved by exercising for 20 to 60 minutes per workout, three to five days per week, at an intensity level between 55–65 percent and 90 percent of the maximum heart rate.[4] Examples of aerobic activities are walking, jogging, stair climbing, cross-country skiing, swimming, rowing, cycling, and sports such as basketball, racquetball, and soccer.

The American Heart Association (AHA) has recognized the importance of physical activity by declaring in 1992 that its opposite, physical inactivity, is a major risk for **cardiovascular diseases**.[5] Further, the AHA stated, "Persons of all ages should include physical activity in a comprehensive program of health promotion and disease prevention." In 1985, The American Cancer Society began recommending exercise to help people protect themselves from cancer.[6] The endorsements of exercise by prestigious organizations such as these came about because of the weight of research evidence.

Trends in Fitness Activities

A compilation of data by the authors of the *Surgeon General's Report on Physical Activity and Health* in 1996 indicated that the most popular leisure-time physical activity by far was walking, followed by gardening or yardwork, stretching exercises, cycling, strength-building exercises, stair climbing, jogging, aerobics, and swimming.

Another analysis of participation in fitness activities and use of fitness equipment between 1987 and 1997 in the United States revealed several trends:[7]

1. Sixty-three percent more people used cardiorespiratory equipment, and 44 percent more used strength-training equipment in 1997 than in 1987.

2. Use of free weights (barbells and dumbbells) rose from 24.5 million participants in 1987 to 43.2 million in 1997; and 39 percent of free-weight users were women.

3. The popularity of treadmills for walking and jogging increased by 720 percent during that time period.

4. Membership in health clubs increased by 63 percent.

5. Purchases of fitness equipment for the home skyrocketed; nearly one-third of all households bought and used exercise equipment during the 10-year period.

6. Baby boomers (now entering their 50s) remain committed to exercise.

7. Participation in high-impact and step aerobics declined, as did low-impact activities such as yoga.

8. Participation in group exercise classes increased.

9. Exercise equipment became more innovative and diversified in an effort to cater to exercise interests.

10. The popularity of personal trainers increased significantly. An estimated 15,000 aspiring exercise professionals took the personal trainer certification exam in 1998 —up from 3,367 in 1992.

A study by the National Sporting Goods Association (NSGA) indicated an increase in exercise participation by older Americans.[8] Participation in seven fitness activities by the 75-and-older age group increased by 27 percent. Participation by the 55- to 64-age group in these activities increased by 17 percent. Contrast that with a 4 percent drop in participation in the 25-to-34 age group. The seven fitness activities in the study were aerobic exercise, cycling, calisthenics, exercise with equipment, exercise walking, jogging, and swimming.

According to the NSGA, 20.4 million women claim to be exercisers, compared to 15.5 million men; and 23 percent of the women exercise regularly, compared to 19 percent for men.[9] Frequency of exercise was defined as participating in physical activity at least twice a week. Two times per week is not enough of an exercise stimulus to improve health significantly, and it is below the American College of Sports Medicine's recommendation for frequency of exercise.

Although the data on the increasing number of older people who exercise are encouraging, the decline in exercise participation for males and females alike as they age indicates that, on the whole, this age group exercises less than all other age groups.[10] People who exercise vigorously and frequently are primarily young adults in the middle and upper socioeconomic strata of U.S. society as defined by income, education, and occupation.

In general, professionals are more active than blue-collar workers in their leisure time. Blue-collar workers as a group, however—particularly those with fewer than 12 years of education—report more on-the-job physical activity than do professionals.[11] The lower-intensity on-the-job expenditure of energy over a 7- to 8-hour day tends to equalize the energy expended by those who participate in structured exercises of higher intensity for 45 to 60 minutes four to five times per week.

A study by the Centers for Disease Control and Prevention in 2001[12] showed no increase in the level of physical activity by Americans since 1990. Approximately 75 percent of American adults reported either no participation in physical activity (28.7 percent) or physical activity below the threshold required to enhance health (45.9 percent).

The exercise movement that began in the late 1960s grew rapidly during the 1970s and continued through the mid-1980s, at which point it slowed and finally plateaued during the 1990s. Annual surveys conducted by Louis Harris and Associates concur with other studies showing that the percentage of Americans who exercise strenuously has not changed significantly during the last 10 years or so.[13] Strenuous exercise was defined as breathing heavily with heart rate and pulse rate accelerated for at least 20 minutes, at least 3 days per week. In spite of the media hype, studies show that today's fitness movement is flat and the majority of Americans are not exercising. One of the many consequences of a sedentary lifestyle is the rising rate of overweight and obesity. Current estimates indicate that 61 percent of adults in the United States are overweight and/or obese.[14]

ACSM and CDC Guidelines

Although physical inactivity is a **risk factor** that crosses all demographic boundaries, the problem is worse for: (a) minority ethnic groups, (b) all people regardless of their ethnicity who are poorly educated, (c) older adults, and (d) people of lower socioeconomic status. **Chronic diseases** such as heart disease, stroke, diabetes, and obesity—all of which respond positively to regular exercise—are most prevalent in these population groups.

Physical inactivity is a risk factor that can be reversed easily and economically. The recommendation for exercise developed jointly by the American College of Sports Medicine (ACSM) and the Centers for Disease Control and Prevention (CDC) for the purpose of health enhancement is that adults should accumulate at least

30 minutes of moderate physical activity over the course of most days (at least 4 days per week).[15] Scientific research has indicated quite clearly that compliance with this modest level of exercise can improve the health of individuals and, concomitantly, the health of the nation.

Furthermore, exercise does not have to be structured or planned, nor must it include the activities associated most with fitness and health—jogging, cycling, rowing, swimming, and the like. Although vigorous activities such as these provide the most benefit, more moderate exercises that contribute to better health include, but are not limited to, everyday physical activities such as mowing the lawn (without a riding mower), gardening, raking leaves, walking, climbing stairs, and washing and waxing the car.

Exercise in a single continuous session is not necessary. A total of 30 minutes of physical activities broken up into three 10-minute bouts is just as effective for health enhancement as one continuous bout. All activities that require some physical exertion should be approached as opportunities for exercise and a bonus for health enhancement even if they must be sprinkled throughout the day. Intermittent low-intensity physical activity spread throughout the day might not improve one's level of physical fitness measurably, but it nevertheless does burn calories. For example, an office worker who spends 2 minutes an hour to send email to co-workers day after day instead of walking down the hall to speak to them personally would gain the energy equivalent of 11 pounds of fat over a decade. This is a substantial weight gain over time from a tiny amount of energy saved.[16]

Add this to all of the other ways at our disposal for saving energy, and we can see that the problem becomes compounded; in 10 years the weight gain is 30 pounds instead of 11. A Scottish researcher estimates that labor-saving devices that affect home life, recreation, and occupation have reduced average energy expenditures in the United Kingdom by 800 calories per day over the last 25 years.

We all can benefit by adopting the philosophy that substituting our own muscle power for mechanically and electronically powered devices is an idea whose time is well past due. When possible, we should walk or bike instead of driving the car, climb stairs instead of using elevators and escalators, take a 10-minute walk instead of a cup of coffee and a doughnut at breaktime, mow our own lawn instead of hiring someone else to do it, and wash our own car instead of running it through the car wash. By taking advantage of these and many other opportunities for physical activity, a person surely will look better and feel better as a result.

Although physical activities such as these are health-enhancing, they may or may not markedly improve physical fitness because most of these activities are performed at only a mild to moderate intensity level. The news is better for those who are willing to exert enough effort to significantly improve their level of physical fitness. A number of studies have shown that the longer people are able to walk or jog during a graded exercise treadmill test, the longer is their life expectancy and the less they are disposed to chronic diseases such as **coronary heart disease** (CHD), cancer, type II diabetes, hypertension, and others.[17,18,19] A substantial improvement in physical fitness is reciprocal in that the more fit people become, the more vigorously they can exercise and the health benefits that accrue are somewhat greater.[20]

Exercise Programs in Business and Industry

Data that are accumulating from work-site exercise programs have provided more ammunition for the physically active life. Many of these programs have been in place long enough to have an impact on employee health. As they attempt to contain the spiraling costs of health care, companies that have invested in worksite health-promotion programs are saving more dollars than they spent initially.

Translating preventive practices into changes in health status takes time and consistent effort. An educational component is necessary to change longstanding behavior patterns such as cigarette smoking, poor nutritional practices, and sedentary living. Time and a sincere commitment are required to control blood pressure and serum levels of cholesterol through lifestyle changes instead of medications.

Data coming from worksite health-promotion programs are encouraging. Companies are discovering that health-care costs are lower, worker absenteeism is down, employee productivity is up, and on-the-job accidents are fewer.[21] Health-promotion programs with physical fitness opportunities either on-site or paid for (partially or fully) by the company are perks to recruit and keep key personnel.

The worksite has great potential for adults to engage in regular physical exercise. In fact, the goals established for worksite fitness programs in *Healthy People 2000*—a national study in which thousands of health professionals contributed to the development of specific national objectives—were exceeded. The more recent *Healthy People 2010* objectives have set worksite fitness goals higher with the expectation that these, too, will be met and exceeded.[22]

The cost of operating a worksite physical fitness program usually can be recovered within a few years. The economic benefits that accrue from quality fitness programs surpass the costs to the company. The latter costs include, among others, professional leadership, facilities, equipment, marketing, and promotion.[23]

The Costs of Sedentary Living

Exercise of moderate intensity, performed consistently, reduces all-cause mortality, increases longevity, and delays or reduces the likelihood of incurring chronic diseases.[24] The most active and most physically fit people have death rates from all causes that are 25 percent to 50 percent lower than those who are least active or least fit.[25] A low level of fitness is one of the most potent risk factors for death from all causes in males, and it is at least as risky as smoking cigarettes.[26] Many of the deaths associated with physical inactivity are premature. The number of lives lost because of inactivity is approximately 250,000 a year.[27] This represents about 12 percent of deaths annually in the United States. Most of these deaths result from coronary heart disease or medical problems such as diabetes and obesity that significantly contribute to CHD.[28] The Johns Hopkins medical editors stated that "when combined with a poor diet, physical inactivity is the second most significant underlying cause of death in the U.S."

Further, exercising regularly delays or reduces the likelihood of succumbing to one or more of the chronic diseases. As a result, active people place less demand on the nation's medical delivery system, and they are more productive occupationally. Conversely, those who choose to lead sedentary lives impose on others the costs associated with their lifestyle.

The financial cost to others (referred to as "external costs") by those who are physically inactive results from payments they receive from collectively financed programs such as health insurance, sick-leave payments, disability insurance, and group life insurance. To finance these programs, active people pay the same premiums and payroll taxes as the sedentary people who are the most frequent users. These programs do not distinguish frequency of utilization, nor do they provide discounts for positive health behaviors. Therefore, they essentially function as social welfare programs that subsidize unhealthy behaviors.

When sedentary people gravitate to an active way of life, everyone benefits. Each minute that people spend walking increases life expectancy by one minute.[29] Because joggers burn calories twice as fast as non-joggers, the former can expect a return of double their exercise time in life expectancy. The Rand Corporation, a well-known California based "think tank," has developed a theoretical model that projects the following: Each mile that a sedentary person walks or jogs will add 21 minutes to that person's life and save society 24 cents in medical and other costs.[30] The economic drain of sedentary living on society is double the external cost associated with cigarette smoking.

Disease and Death Patterns

The fitness movement developed largely as a reaction to innovations in medicine, science, and technology and their relationship to the changing patterns of disease and death patterns in the United States. **Communicable diseases** (tuberculosis, pneumonia, typhoid fever, smallpox, scarlet fever, and others) were the leading causes of death during the early years of the 20th century.

Advances in medical science have virtually eradicated these maladies and threats to life, but they have been replaced by chronic **degenerative diseases** such as heart disease, stroke, cancer, diabetes, and the like. This group of diseases, largely lifestyle-induced, has reached epidemic proportions. Many authorities refer to these diseases as voluntary or self-inflicted, thereby emphasizing the influence of negative choices and unhealthy behaviors on the development and course of these diseases.

Approximately 58,000,000 people in the United States have one or more forms of cardiovascular disease.[31] Cardiovascular diseases accounts for approximately 39 percent of all deaths in the United States, about 950,000 deaths annually. About half of these deaths (500,000) are the result of coronary heart disease. Although most Americans are aware of this type of heart disease, most people don't fully understand the behaviors necessary to prevent or delay it. The Framingham Heart Study—a landmark study of heart disease—identified the risk factors connected with heart disease. This ongoing study began in 1949 and continues to this day, turning out valuable information from the subjects they began studying decades ago.

As risk factors were identified, the realization evolved that heart disease was not the inevitable consequence of aging but, instead, an acquired disease that is potentially preventable. Cigarette smoking, high blood pressure, elevated levels of blood fats, diabetes, overweight, stress, lack of exercise, and a family history of heart disease were found to be highly related to heart attack and stroke. Most of these risk factors can be modified by the way we live.

Within our control are opportunities to choose what to eat and how much, whether to smoke cigarettes, whether to exercise, and how to control stress. We can choose when to be screened for blood pressure and blood fats, and we can choose whether to act upon that information. During the last four decades, millions of Americans have changed their eating, smoking, and exercise habits. Consequently, deaths from cardiovascular disease declined by approximately 51 percent during this time.[32] Even though other factors are involved in this favorable trend, modifications in lifestyle have made a significant contribution.

Life today is considerably different from life in the early 1900s. Scientific and technological advances have made us functionally mechanized. Labor-saving devices proliferate in all facets of life—occupation, home life, and leisure-time pursuits—and always with the promise of more and better to come. Each new invention has helped to foster a receptive attitude toward a life of ease, and we have become accustomed to the easy way of doing things. The mechanized way is usually the most expedient way, and in our time-oriented society, this has become another stimulus to indulge in the sedentary lifestyle.

Today, exercise for fitness is programmed into our lives as an entity separate from our other functions. In contrast, the energy expenditures of our forebears were integrated into their work, play, and home life. Physical fitness was necessary, and fit people were the rule rather than the exception. Tilling the soil, digging ditches, and working in factories were physically demanding jobs. Lumberjack contests and square dances were vigorous leisure pursuits. Being a wife and taking care of home and family required long hours doing arduous tasks. In the early years of the twentieth century, one-third of the energy for operating factories came from muscle power. By 1970, this figure had dropped to less than 1 percent, reflecting the declining energy demand of our jobs.

The turn of the twentieth century found 70 percent of the population working long, hard hours to produce food. Children of this era walked several miles to school and did chores when they returned home. Today, only 3 percent of the population, using highly mechanized equipment, are involved in the production of food, and their children ride in motor vehicles to school. Adults drive to the store, circle the parking lot to get as close as possible to the entrance, and ride elevators and escalators while there. We mow the lawn with a riding mower, rely on a cart when we play golf, wash dishes and clothes in appropriate appliances, change television channels with a remote control, and open garage doors in the same manner.

These are simply observations of life in the United States. This is not to imply that the fruits of science and technology should be repudiated but, rather, that the results and their impact upon us be viewed in perspective and acted upon accordingly. Inventions of the Industrial Age have significantly reduced the level of physical activity required to earn a living. Machines and automation have taken much of the physical labor out of our occupations. And now we find ourselves moving at the speed of light into the Information Age, with its potential for further reducing the need for physical activity. Cell phones, faxes, electronic mail, and the proliferation of computers for business and home have changed the way we do business and access information—and all of this is accomplished while we sit down.[33]

The leisure-time activities of young people 10 to 17 years of age also have changed. Computerized games, video games, and television watching have replaced more active leisure-time games and activities. These sedentary pursuits seem to be contributing to the rise in obesity in this age group in the United States today. One study found that at least 25 percent of U.S. children spend 4 hours or more viewing television daily.[34] Reducing TV viewing time by just 3 hours per week and converting those hours to moderately intense physical activity would improve physical fitness and health status for this age group.

Futurists of the 1960s predicted that technology would take over many of the laborious tasks in the workplace as well as the home. The result of all of this would be a substantial reduction in the time required to earn a living and to manage the household, leaving us with an abundance of free time. Obviously this prediction was off the mark and has not materialized for much of the population. At that time, the expectation was that the new technology would enable the workforce to do the work in less time, and this ultimately would lead to a 4-day workweek.

In reality, the new technology enabled U.S. workers to do more work in the same amount of time, thereby increasing productivity while expending less energy. As corporations have downsized, fewer workers using modern technology and working longer hours are more productive than the full workforce used to be.

Managing Time

All of the changes over the past century have made it difficult to find time to schedule exercise. Effective management of time is becoming more important as we attempt to balance work, leisure activity, and sleep in a 24-hour day. To commit the time and effort required to exercise consistently, we must understand its relevance to a healthy life.

Effective time managers are skilled in identifying and prioritizing goals. They identify the ultimate objective and then set realistic short-term goals that are attainable with sustained effort. The goals that are established should be specific to allow evaluation of progress. Finally, goals should be accompanied by a timeline for accomplishments.

Wise time managers use a variety of tools to help them accomplish their daily tasks. For example, many people generate a list of things to do for each day. They carry the list with them on a 3×5 index card or pocket-size notebook and cross off the tasks as they are completed during the day.

Another useful tool is a weekly or monthly calendar containing the fixed items that remain the same every week, such as classes, work, meals, and meetings. Also included are important nonfixed items such as tests, due dates for written and oral assignments, and vacation. Filling out a calendar like this indicates pockets of time available for physical activity, study, and other pursuits. When total time is examined systematically, it is surprising how much time is left over.

As important as time availability is, people still must be motivated to use it constructively. A national survey conducted among "less active" Americans indicated that 84 percent watched television a minimum of 3 hours per week.[35] This suggests that they have leisure time available but would rather watch television than participate in physical activity. Television viewing is running into stiff competition from another sedentary pursuit—the home computer—and this is compounding the difficulty of finding time for physical activities.

Rationale for Choosing Walking and Jogging

Although people have inhabited the Earth for many centuries, only during the last 75 years have such drastic changes in lifestyle been generated. At the same time, our basic need for physical activity has not changed. Our bodies were constructed for, and thrive on, physical work, but we find ourselves thrust into the automobile, television, and sofa age, and we simply have not had enough time to adapt to this new, sedentary way of living. Perhaps 100,000 years from now the sedentary life will be the healthy life. At this stage of our development, though, the law of use and disuse continues to prevail: That which is used becomes stronger, and that which is not used becomes weaker. For simple verification of this physiological principle, witness a leg removed from a cast after 8 weeks and note the atrophy of the limb.

Many people, myself included, believe that our new ways of living are precipitating, or at least significantly contributing to, the diseases that are affecting modern affluent humankind. These ways of living are unique to highly industrialized nations. By contrast, the underdeveloped nations, with their different lifestyles, do not experience this phenomenon to the same extent.

Before developing or engaging in any form of physical exercise program, beginners should determine what their expectations are. What goals, both short- and long-term, do you wish to achieve? Identifying goals will guide you regarding how hard, how often, how long, and what activities will comprise your exercise program. Once you resolve these questions, you can tailor the program to meet your specific objectives. If you follow through, you will have a high probability of success.

The choice to walk, jog, or combine the two as the activity mode by which to attain health and fitness objectives has a significant base of support in research. Both activities are effective and popular.

Identifying goals will guide you regarding how hard, how often, how long, and what activities will comprise your exercise program.

Walking

For human beings, walking is the natural form of locomotion. It is a low-risk, low-impact activity that can be done almost anywhere, by almost anybody (including many who have disabilities), in most environments, and within a reasonable timeframe.

Walking uses a heel-to-toe motion so the foot strike at landing is at the heel and the push-off is at the end of the big toe. This action dissipates the force of impact with the ground over the widest possible foot area. The foot rolling forward generates horizontal momentum for forward movement. The advancing foot lands before the rear foot leaves the ground, ensuring that one foot is always in contact with the ground. Forward motion of this type minimizes the impact of landing.

For beginners, walking is an effective introduction to physical activity. Walking can be manipulated to meet a variety of objectives. In addition to being an entry point into exercise, it can be a lead-up conditioner for other types of activity. Or it can be the end product for developing and maintaining physical fitness. This can be accomplished through brisk walking or variations such as speed walking, power walking, and race walking.

Millions of people are walking for health and fitness. More than 10,000 walking events are held annually. These include walk-a-thons, fun walks, and competitive race walks. More than 6,500 walking clubs are scattered throughout the country. Some of these feature hiking and orienteering (using a map and compass to find the path between two land marks).

Slow walking speeds produce substantial health benefits but result in a minimal increase in fitness level. Higher speeds result in improvements in both health and fitness. In one study, women subjects were divided into three groups of different walking intensity.[36] One group walked at 3 miles per hour (mph) ("strollers"), a second group walked at 4 mph ("brisk walkers"), and the last group walked at 5 mph ("aerobic walkers"). The subjects walked 3 miles per day, 5 days per week. At the end of 24 weeks, the data were analyzed. The results indicated that physical fitness improved on a dose-response basis: The fastest walking group improved the most, and the slowest walking group improved the least. The risk of cardiovascular disease was reduced equally among the three groups. The 3-mph walkers benefited as much as the fastest walkers with regard to favorably changing the cardiovascular risk profile.

Data collected from more than 72,000 nurses showed a strong inverse (or negative) association between walking and the risk for coronary heart disease.[37] The women who walked briskly or regularly participated in other vigorous aerobic exercises had substantial reductions in the incidence of coronary events compared to women who were primarily sedentary. If enhancement of health is the major objective of exercise, walking—even slow walking—fits the bill nicely. If, however, the major objective is to improve physical fitness, fast walking is a satisfactory activity. The bonus for those who engage in exercise for the purpose of fitness is that they achieve the health benefits simultaneously.

Jogging

Jogging is a higher impact activity than walking. Jogging requires that both feet must be off the ground for a split-second during every stride. Because joggers become airborne, their impact with the ground is greater and the expenditure of energy is higher than that of walking except under two circumstances.

1. The energy expenditure or oxygen cost of very slow jogging (5 mph) is equal to walking at the same speed. At speeds faster than 5 mph, the oxygen cost of walking exceeds that of jogging because of the in-efficiency associated with very fast walking.

2. The oxygen cost of jogging up a hill is about half that of walking up the same hill at the same speed. Both feet come off the ground during jogging, so some of the vertical lift needed to run up the hill occurs naturally, thereby lowering the net cost of the vertical work.

Some surfaces are better than others. Still, jogging can be pursued almost anywhere that is devoid of hazards such as potholes or jutting rocks. Jogging also is time-effective. For instance, a person might take 1 hour to walk 4 miles but only 35 to 40 minutes to slow-jog the same distance. The savings in time is important to many busy people.

Even though the popularity of jogging has declined somewhat in the last few years, it nonetheless remains alive and kicking. An estimated 20 million people jog a minimum of three times per week. Studies have shown that joggers as a whole are highly dedicated to this activity and are compliant exercisers. Jogging will remain an effective means of improving health and fitness and likely will continue to appeal to a large number of participants.

A factor that contributes to the appeal of walking and jogging is that these activities can be done either indoors or outdoors and in most environmental conditions. From the perspective of clothing and equipment needs, a good pair of shoes is mandatory to protect against potential injury. The environmental conditions should dictate the remainder of the attire.

Another appealing factor is that participants can walk or jog alone or with others. Walking or jogging in solitude provides the opportunity for introspection, or to mentally organize that paper that you have to write for class, or it provides a setting for the mind to roam freely. Walking or jogging also offers the opportunity for socialization and camaraderie with friends who are interested in the same form of exercise, and it is an ideal circumstance for conversation.

Health-Related Fitness

The primary purposes of health-related exercise are the prevention of disease and the attainment of well-being. This can be achieved by consistent participation in mild to moderately vigorous aerobic activities. The components of **health-related fitness** are:

1. **Cardiorespiratory endurance**, the maximum ability to take in, deliver, and extract oxygen for physical work

2. **Muscular strength**, the maximum amount of force that a muscle or group of muscles can exert in a single contraction

3. **Muscle endurance**, the capacity to exert repetitive muscular force

4. **Flexibility**, the range of movement around the joints of the body

5. **Body composition**, the amount of fat versus lean tissue in the body.

Attaining aerobic physical fitness requires individuals to exercise vigorously enough to improve their cardio-respiratory endurance and muscle

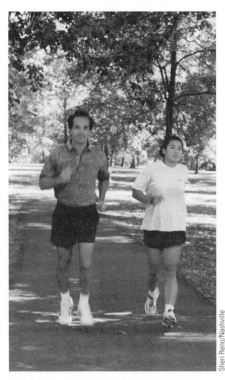

A person can walk or jog alone or with someone else.

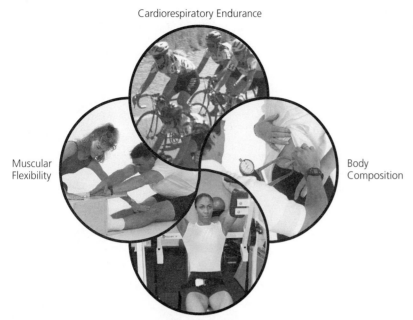

Cardiorespiratory Endurance

Muscular Flexibility

Body Composition

Muscular Strength and Endurance

Health-related components of physical fitness.

Muscular Strength and Endurance photo by Kristin Dilworth. All other photos © Fitness & Wellness, Inc. Reprinted by permission.

are not mutually exclusive. Some individuals perform in athletic contests as a means by which to meet their health-related goals. A competitor in an endurance event is developing health-related components even though the major goal is performance-related. A perceived lack of athletic ability should not be a barrier to exercise for health enhancement because many health-related activities require little athletic ability. Walking and jogging are prime examples.

Terms

Aerobic exercise	Degenerative
Body composition	diseases
Cardiorespiratory	Flexibility
endurance	Health-related
Cardiovascular	fitness
diseases	Muscle endurance
Chronic diseases	Muscular strength
Communicable	Performance-
diseases	related fitness
Coronary heart	Risk factor
disease	

endurance. Exercises for the development and maintenance of physical fitness increase the energy level and enhance physical appearance. A standard for aerobic fitness is to exercise 5 days per week, for approximately 45 minutes per exercise session, at an intensity level of 70 percent to 80 percent of the maximum heart rate (discussed in Chapter 3).

Performance-Related Fitness

Performance-related fitness requires the abilities necessary for proficient execution of sports skills. Although these abilities are not necessary to enhance health, they are indispensable to those who participate competitively in physical activities. The performance-related components are speed, power, balance, coordination, agility, and reaction time. Successful performance in games such as racquetball, tennis, basketball, volleyball, and badminton—to name a few—is dependent upon these athletic abilities.

The health-related and performance-related components

Summary

❖ Most people in the United States do not exercise often enough or vigorously enough to improve their health.

❖ The exercise movement has plateaued in the last few years despite compelling evidence that exercise is necessary for health and wellness.

❖ Mechanization, the product of science and technology, has removed much of the labor from our occupations, homes, and leisure-time activities.

❖ The American Heart Association has declared physical inactivity as a major risk factor for heart disease.

❖ Less than one-fourth of adults in the United States are exercising at the level recommended for heart health.

❖ Physical inactivity is more prevalent among (a) minority groups, (b) poorly educated people, (c) older adults, and (d) those in the lower socioeconomic levels.

❖ For health enhancement, the American College of Sports Medicine recommends participation in mild to moderate physical activity for at least 30 minutes 4 days a week.

❖ Everyday activities such as walking, climbing stairs, mowing the lawn, raking leaves, and similar activities contribute to health.

❖ A person doesn't have to exercise in one continuous session; it can be done at various times during the day.

❖ Fitness and wellness worksite programs are cutting the cost of health care as a result of less absenteeism, greater productivity, and fewer on-the-job accidents.

❖ Consistent participation in exercise reduces the risk of death from all causes.

❖ People who have a sedentary lifestyle receive more payments from health insurance, disability insurance, and group life insurance, and they take more sick leave than physically active people.

❖ The Rand Corporation has estimated that each mile a sedentary person walks or jogs will add 21 minutes to that person's life and save society 24 cents in medical and other costs.

❖ Risk factors for heart disease, identified by researchers who participated in the Framingham Study, are cigarette smoking, high blood pressure and blood fats, diabetes, overweight, stress, lack of exercise, and a family history of heart disease.

❖ The death rate from cardiovascular disease has declined by more than 50 percent in the last four decades.

❖ The workweek has been on the increase during the decades of the 1980s and 1990s.

❖ As leisure time decreases, time-management skills assume greater importance as we attempt to balance work and play.

❖ Walking for exercise is a low-risk, low-impact activity that can be done in most environments and can satisfy the needs of beginners and experienced exercisers alike.

❖ Walking can enhance health and develop aerobic fitness.

❖ Jogging is a higher impact activity than walking; it uses more energy and requires more oxygen under most conditions.

❖ At approximately 5 mph, the oxygen cost of walking is equal to that of jogging.

❖ Walking up hills requires more oxygen than jogging up the same hills at the same speed.

❖ Walking and jogging can be done indoors or outdoors.

❖ A quality pair of shoes is the only equipment or special clothing necessary for walkers and joggers.

❖ Walking and jogging contribute to the health-related fitness components: cardiorespiratory endurance, muscular strength and endurance, flexibility, and body composition.

❖ The components of performance-related fitness are speed, power, coordination, agility, balance, and reaction time.

Notes

1. National Center for Chronic Disease Prevention and Health Promotion, *Physical Activity and Health: A Report of the Surgeon General* (Atlanta: Centers for Disease Control and Prevention, 1996).
2. "American's Health Priorities Not in Line with Practices," *Fitness Management*, 17(6):8, May, 2001.
3. Cited in "Portion Distortion," *Tufts University Health and Nutrition Letter*, 18(12):4–5, February, 2001.
4. ACSM, *ACSM's Guidelines for Exercise Testing and Prescription* (Philadelphia: Lippincott Williams and Wilkins, 2000).
5. "It's Official: Inactivity Increases Coronary Risks," *Harvard Health Letter*, 3:3 (1992), 8.

6. *Cancer Facts and Figures 1992* (Atlanta: American Cancer Society, 1997).

7. *Tracking the Fitness Movement, 1987–1997: A Decade of Change* (North Palm Beach, FL: Fitness Products Council, 1998).

8. "Older Adults and Women Exercise the Most," *Fitness Management*, 14:11 (Oct. 1998), 8–10.

9. Fitness Management, Note 8.

10. D. C. Nieman, *Exercise Testing and Prescription A Health-Related Approach* (Mountain View, CA: Mayfield, 1999).

11. P. C. Wagener, *Health Conditions Among the Currently Employed: United States, 1988* (National Center for Health Statistics, Series 10, No. 186 (PHS) 93-1412) (Washington, DC: U. S. Government Printing Office, 1993).

12. "Most U. S. Adults Are Sedentary," *Fitness Management*, 17(6): 8–11, 2001.

13. T. Dybdahl, *The Prevention Index '97: A Report Card on the Nation's Health* (Emmaus, PA: Rodale Press, 1997).

14. Portion Distortion, Note 3.

15. R. R. Pate, M. Pratt, S. N. Blair, et al. "Physical Activity and Public Health: A Recommendation from the Centers for Disease Control and Prevention and the American College of Sports Medicine," *Journal of the American Medical Association*, 273 (1995), 402–407.

16. B. Liebman, "Take a Hike." Interview with Steve Blair, *Nutrition Action Healthletter*, 26:1 (Jan./Feb., 1999), 1–7.

17. Liebman, Note 15.

18. M. Fenton, "Walking Weighs In," *Walking Magazine*, 16(5):98, July/August, 2001.

19. S. N. Blair, J. B. Kampert, H. W. Kohl, et al., "Influences of Cardiorespiratory Fitness and Other Resources on Cardiovascular Disease and All-Cause Mortality in Men and Women," *Journal of the American Medical Association*, 276: 205–210; 1996.

20. S. N. Blair, H. W. Kohl, C. E. Barlow et al., "Changes in Physical Fitness and All-Cause Mortality: A Prospective Study of Healthy and Unhealthy Men," *Journal of the American Medical Association*, 273: 1093–1098, 1995.

21. C. G. Spain, and B. D. Franks, "Healthy People 2010: Physical Activity and Fitness," *PCPFS Research Digest*, 3(13): 1–16, March, 2001.

22. Blair, Kohl, Barlow, et al., Note 20.

23. U. S. Dept. of Health and Human Services, *Healthy People 2010 Objectives* (Washington, DC: U. S. Government Printing Office, 2000).

24. J. C. Erfurt, A. Foote, M. A. Heirich, and B. M. Rock, *The Wellness Outreach at Work Program: A Step-by-Step Guide* (NIH Publication No. 95–3043) (Washington DC: National Institute of Health, Aug. 1995).

25. I. M. Lee and R. S. Paffenbarger, "Do Physical Activity and Physical Fitness Avert Premature Mortality?" *Exercise and Sport Science Reviews*, 24: 135–169, 1996.

26. Blair, Kampert, Kohl, Note 19.

27. L. H. Kushi, R. M. Fee, and A. R. Folsom et al., "Physical Activity and Mortality in Postmenopausal Women," *Journal of the American Medical Association*, 227: 1287–1292, 1997.

28. Johns Hopkins Medical Staff, "Tapping into the "Real" Fountain of Youth," *Health After 50*, 13(6): 4–5, 7, Aug 2001.

29. Lee, Paffenbarger, Note 25.

30. Lee, Paffenbarger, Note 25.

31. American Heart Association, *1999 Heart and Stroke Statistical Update* (Dallas: AHA, 1998).

32. American Heart Association, *Heart and Stroke Facts* (Dallas: AHA, 1999).

33. W. Haskill, "Physical Activity, Sport, and Health: Toward the Next Century," *Research Quarterly for Exercise and Sport*, 67 (Supplement to No. 3) (Sept. 1996), 537–547.

34. R. E. Anderson, et al. "Relationship of Physical Activity and Television Watching with Body Weight and Level of Fatness Among Children: Results from Third National Health and Nutrition Examination Survey," *Journal of the American Medical Association*, 229: 938–942, 1998.

35. "Most Less Active Americans Want to be More Active," *NASPE News*, Winter 1994, p. 11.

36. J. J. Duncan, et al., "Women Walking for Health and Fitness," *Journal of the American Medical Association*, 266, 1991, p. 3295.

37. J. E. Manson, et al., "A Prospective Study of Walking as Compared with Vigorous Exercise in the Prevention of Coronary Heart Disease in Women," *New England Journal of Medicine*, 341(1): 650–658, Aug. 26, 1999.

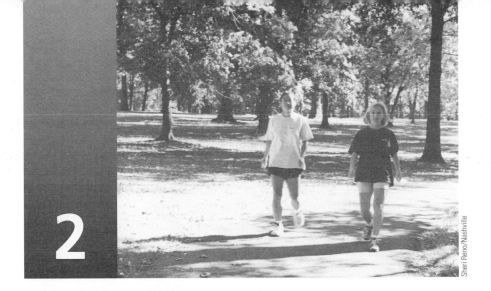

Sheri Reno/Nashville

Motivation and Motivational Techniques

Outline

Motivating people to begin and maintain an active way of life is a formidable and perplexing task. Although much has been said and written about the value of exercise, only 22 percent of people living in the United States are active enough to improve their health status.[1] After three decades into the exercise movement, the majority of Americans are still essentially sedentary. Some are not convinced of the value of exercise. Others are unaware of its value. Still others simply prefer to be sedentary.

Moving Toward an Active Lifestyle

Motivating people to begin exercising is indeed difficult, and keeping them exercising after they begin is even more difficult. The exercise dropout rate is 50 percent during the initial 6 months.[2] Most of these people discontinue their exercise programs during the first 3 months,[3] and 70 percent to 80 percent drop out before the end of the first year.[4] Changing behavior is a complex phenomenon. Though many theories and models seek to explain and describe the process, scientists still are unable to predict with a high degree of accuracy who will succeed. No single theory or model will work for everyone because each individual is unique, with unique circumstances and needs. The models are not all-encompassing, and all of the factors involved in behavior change have yet to be identified.

Most young children are fairly active, but studies have shown that their level of activity declines by approximately 50 percent during their progression through the school years.[5] Children seem to react primarily to parental influence regarding physical activity. If parents exercise regularly and value the physically active life, their children most likely will emulate them. Conversely, sedentary parents who do not value physical activity often rear children who reflect similar attitudes and behavior patterns.

At the secondary school level, classmates, friends, and peer groups seem to exert the most influence upon behaviors.[6] A supportive environment for the active life is created when an adolescent identifies with a peer group that appreciates and participates in physical activities. The opposite occurs if the peer group devalues physical activity.

Peer groups exert the most influence on the attitudes and behaviors of college-age people.[7] Most middle-aged and elderly adults respond well to support from a spouse, friends, co-workers, and health professionals, particularly physicians.

Components of Behavior Change

Research has suggested that exercise and physical activities consist of behaviors that are more complex than other health-related behaviors.[8] Although exercise has some commonalities with other health behaviors, it is inherently unique. Researchers continue to attempt to develop a model of behavior applicable to exercise that will enable them to identify potential dropouts as well as individ-

uals who will persevere. If potential dropouts can be identified early, they can be targeted for appropriate intervention that might increase the probability of their adhering to an exercise regimen.

One of the personality traits associated with adherence to exercise is **self-motivation**, the desire to persist at a task without constant help or praise. Exercisers in this category tend to (a) set short-term goals that are attainable, (b) select activities they enjoy, (c) keep the workout manageable in terms of time and effort required, and (d) join a group for a portion or the entirety of a workout.[9]

The reasons that exercise dropouts offer most often are lack of time, inconvenient or inaccessible exercise site, work conflicts, and poor spousal support.[10] They also cite situational factors, such as the travel requirements of their jobs, as impediments to regular participation.

Determining whether these barriers to exercise are actual or perceived is difficult. Those who adhere to exercise often live farther away from the exercise facility and have no more leisure time than dropouts do. Support from mates repeatedly has been shown to be a predictor of adherence to exercise, but some adherents indicate that it is less important than other factors. Perhaps one of the differences between those who continue to exercise and those who don't is that the dropouts perceive impediments to exercise as real barriers. Adherents perceive these same barriers as mere inconveniences that they can easily surmount. Turning dropouts into adherents, therefore, might be accomplished by changing dropouts' perceptions. Providing instruction in time management and flexible exercise hours and developing home exercise programs for these people might be productive.

Some generalizations regarding adherence to exercise are as follows:[11]

1. Blue-collar workers, smokers, the elderly and obese people are less likely to begin and sustain exercise

in either a supervised or an individual program.

2. People who are highly self-motivated are more likely to continue unsupervised exercise.

3. Perceptions of lack of time and inconvenience lead to dropping out, but some exercisers continue despite the same barriers.

4. Reinforcement from health and exercise professionals, particularly physicians, support from significant others, feelings of well-being, and attainment of goals seem to be important factors in continuation of exercise.

Learning theories indicate that the assimilation of new and complicated patterns of behaviors, such as moving from a sedentary lifestyle to a more active one, might require an incremental approach to attain the desired behavior.[12] For example, if the long-range goal is to walk 45 minutes a day, the person might begin with 15-minute daily walks. When the exerciser adjusts and becomes comfortable with this level of energy expenditure, 5 minutes could be added each week to the daily walk until achieving the target. At this point the exerciser might be satisfied to continue this level of exercise for a lifetime (maintenance) or might establish a different, more difficult goal. The success associated with accomplishing the first goal will contribute to attaining the second.

Adhering to the program depends substantially on the reinforcement or rewards received from participating in exercise. Rewards can take many forms. A reward can be **extrinsic** (external) **reinforcement** or **intrinsic** (internal) **reinforcement**, or it might have physical parameters. Receiving praise and encouragement from others for example, are extrinsic rewards. Extrinsic rewards are necessary during the first few months of the exercise program because they help to shape and establish the exercise habit.[13]

After a couple of months of regular participation, intrinsic rewards become more important, and eventually

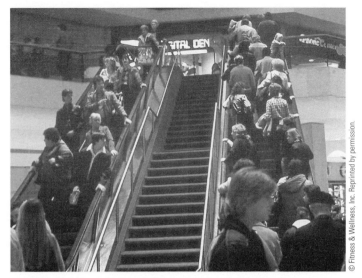
People would benefit from taking stairs instead of escalators.

become the primary reinforcer because at this point the exerciser begins to experience some of the physiological and emotional benefits associated with consistent effort. A feeling of accomplishment for reaching a goal that required commitment and effort is an intrinsic reward. Examples of the physical benefits that result from exercise are a gain in muscle, loss of fat, and an increase in energy. Any or all of these forms of **positive feedback** can provide the incentive and motivation for persisting in the program.[14] The new exercise behavior, which requires time and effort to sustain, will have to compete with or replace former sedentary behaviors that also were satisfying and rewarding, such as watching television and "surfing the net."

The ultimate goal is to participate consistently in deliberately conceived physical activities such as jogging, cycling, rowing, cross-country skiing, swimming, weight training, and the like. On the way to achieving this goal, we should take advantage of the opportunities in daily life to increase the level and frequency of our energy expenditure by mowing the lawn, washing and waxing the car by hand, taking the stairs instead of escalators and elevators, walking instead of driving, and many other activities.

Changing Health Behavior: Nationwide Efforts

In an effort to get Americans moving more, public and private efforts alike have promoted the benefits of engaging in physical activity. Among these are an anti-smoking TV campaign, a seminal Surgeon General's report, a CDC program, and a NASPE public service announcement.

Electronic Media Campaigns

The electronic media—television in particular—have been used successfully on occasion to change health behavior. Two decades ago the tobacco companies were advertising their products heavily through TV during a time when sales were robust and increasing. The commercials were glitzy, glamorous, sexy, and targeted to teenagers and young adults.

In response to pressure from health professionals and other concerned citizens regarding the proliferation of smoking ads on television with no rebuttal, Congress enacted a fairness doctrine, or equal-time law, compelling the television industry to provide time for anti-smoking commercials. Within 2 short years cigarette sales declined significantly. The result was that the tobacco companies voluntarily removed all tobacco ads from TV.

This chain of events worked in the tobacco companies' favor in that:

1. Cigarette sales increased the year after the ads were removed.
2. The equal-time concept was nullified, so the anti-smoking commercials dried up as well.

The tobacco companies transferred their advertising dollars to various forms of the print media and sponsorship of sporting events, and the anti-smoking messages had no place to go. The point of the story is that people who watch television sometimes do act upon what they are exposed to.

Surgeon General's Report

In July 1996, the Surgeon General's report, on the importance of physical activity for improving health, preventing disease, and increasing longevity, was released amid a great deal of fanfare. TV newscasters introduced the report nationally and locally. It was discussed on TV news magazine shows and on morning news and entertainment shows. This report extolled the virtues of *moderate* physical activity. Vigorous exercise, which produces even better results, is not necessary to improve health. Activities that are a part of daily living can enhance health if these are done at an intensity level equal to walking 3 to 4 miles per hour.

This message should have resonated with the public. Instead, it generated about as much interest and excitement as announcing that "the sky is blue." It is disappointing that the public showed so little response to the Surgeon General's report.

National Surveys

One year after the Surgeon General's report was issued, the National Coalition for Promoting Physical Activity commissioned a national survey regarding the public's knowledge of physical activity and its benefits.[15] Some of the highlights were:

1. Only one-third of those surveyed were aware of the Surgeon General's report.
2. More than half were unaware that exercise has a cumulative effect, that it can be dispersed throughout the day and still produce health benefits.
3. At least 25 percent stated that they would *like* to be more active.
4. More than one-third are marginally active, a level that is not active enough to improve health.

A nationally sponsored survey commissioned by the editors of *Parade Magazine* found that half of Americans do not exercise, but 87 percent of them said they should.[16] Commenting on the U. S. lifestyle,

Nancy Dickey, President Elect of the American Medical Association, said, "In terms of awareness and knowing about good health, I'd give Americans an A-minus or B-plus. But in terms of doing what we know we should, most of us—myself included—deserve only a C or a C-minus."

If we could distill into pill form the physiological, health, psychological, and emotional benefits derived from exercise, Americans would line up and pay any reasonable amount of money to get it. Yet, all of these benefits are there for the taking if we are willing to devote the time and effort to get them.

CDC Program

In an effort to inform and motivate Americans to become active, the Centers for Disease Control and Prevention (CDC) developed a program entitled "Physical Activity: It's Everywhere You Go." The program and its materials (three manuals, television messages from Olympic speed skater Dan Jansen, ads, and posters) were designed for health professionals and community leaders to effectively spread the word at the grassroots level.

NASPE Promotion

The National Association for Sport and Physical Education (NASPE) developed 30-second and 60-second public service announcements for television, to educate the public about the importance of developing and delivering quality physical education programs in the public schools.[17] Former Surgeon General C. Everett Koop showed his support for this effort by signing the cover letter that was sent to 210 TV stations throughout the United States.

Time will tell whether these initiatives and others like them will be successful. Despite a strong message from some of the most prestigious and influential health agencies and individuals in the country, the public might not act upon it. Although attaining knowledge is a necessary first step, it does not necessarily result in action.

Transtheoretical Model

One interesting theory of the process of behavior change is the **transtheoretical model**.[18] The five stages in this model are:

1. *Precontemplation*. Applied to exercise, individuals at this first stage are not exercising. They probably are not considering exercising, and they might be denying that exercise should be part of their lifestyle. People in this stage need a solid reason to change their behavior. One approach is to encourage them to move slowly along the continuum of stages instead of attempting to thrust themselves directly into the action stage.[19] Understanding why physical activity is important—that it promotes health enhancement and an improved quality of life—leads to the next stage.

2. *Contemplation*. Knowledge, or some other motivator such as "It's time to lose a few pounds" or "My 48-year-old neighbor died of a heart attack this morning and I'm his age," could be stimulus enough for an individual to seriously consider starting an exercise program. When this happens, the individual has progressed to the contemplation stage.

3. *Preparation*. At this stage the person demonstrates some overt movement signaling an intent to exercise, such as purchasing fitness equipment or a pair of walking/running shoes or joining a health club.

4. *Action*. The person finally arrives at this stage when he or she actually becomes involved in some physical activity.

5. *Maintenance*. If the behavior change is successful, the person adheres to the program for some time. Even so, people backslide for various reasons, and some drop out even after they have participated for a long time.

The time a person spends in any stage varies, and he or she might move

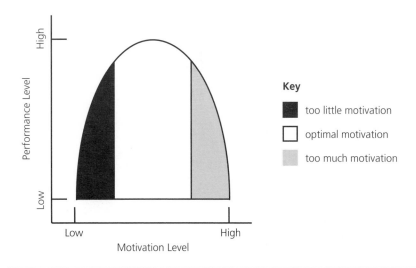

Figure 2.1 Inverted U hypothesis.

back and forth among the stages. Although this model provides a framework for changing behavior, it does not work for all people, nor does it assure that a person will sustain the new behavior. People who drop out or backslide, however, can take comfort in the fact that the more attempts they make to establish a behavior change—in this case, lifetime exercise—the greater is the probability of eventual success.

Inverted U Hypothesis

Some psychologists have determined that a moderate level of motivation is optimal. Too little is likely to result in early failure, and too much may result in injury and burnout. In either case, when motivation is affected adversely, adherence to exercise wanes and the program, with all its good intentions and potential benefits, is terminated. This is graphically depicted by the inverted U hypothesis in Figure 2.1.

Fitness: A Lifelong Commitment

Even the best laid plans sometimes go awry, and forces beyond our control interfere with the exercise program. Injuries and illnesses, job responsibilities, job-related travel, family and other obligations could interrupt your exercise program. If exercise is truly a

priority in your life, though, you can surmount these barriers and find the time and the means to resume exercise.

To avert this all-too-familiar scenario, we should approach our health and fitness goals slowly and patiently, albeit progressively. We must learn to contain our enthusiasm so as not to attempt too much too soon during the early phases of the program. Physical fitness is not achieved after only 2 weeks of frenetic training. Developing and maintaining physical fitness is a lifelong endeavor. It requires a sizable commitment of time and effort, but the results are eminently worthwhile. You supply the time and effort, and this text will provide you with the necessary knowledge. Appropriate application of these ingredients will increase your likelihood of success.

Factors that are motivating to one person may not have the same effect upon another person because of differences in experience, interests, aims, objectives, intelligence, and many other factors. Therefore, selecting the precise factors that will motivate any given individual to participate in a long-term walking or jogging program is conjectural at best.

Most people become involved with exercise for health-related reasons such as to lose weight, reduce stress and anxiety, prevent or delay heart disease, increase muscle strength, sleep more restfully, or live better and longer. The initial reason for participation often becomes the primary reinforcer for maintaining the program. In some instances the original reason is blended with others or assumes lesser importance as the person progresses and new goals assume greater priority.

Some Motivational Techniques

Various strategies are available that may motivate us to exercise. Predicting the precise motive that will stimulate a specific individual to exercise, how-ever, remains elusive. The following are practical suggestions to help people begin and continue an exercise program. Not every suggestion will appeal to every person. Still, one or more of these ideas might stimulate you toward a lifestyle that includes exercise.

1. *Develop a knowledge base.* Understanding the need for exercise, as well as the associated health-related benefits, is a sufficient stimulus for some people to act. Ken Cooper's first book motivated millions of seden-tary Americans to become physically active.[20] Knowledge provides a ration-ale for an active life, and for those who respond positively to cognitive information, it might be a key motivator.

For many people, however, knowl-edge about the beneficial health effects of exercise usually is not enough of a motivator. Even though most people know that exercise is good for their health, most don't participate. Knowledge is simply not sufficient to stimulate most people to make positive behavioral changes. For instance, millions of people know that smoking cigarettes is harmful to their health, yet they continue to smoke. Other motivators are needed.

2. *Set realistic goals.* Goals for exercise should be specific and attain-able. They should address the major accomplishments you will attempt to achieve. Goals might be to control weight, develop muscles, increase energy reserves, manage stress, reduce serum cholesterol or blood pressure, prevent chronic disease, or compete in road races. Walking and jogging, or a combination of the two, are effective exercise modalities for achieving all of these goals.

Novices might walk for 20 to 30 minutes per day, four or five days per week. Beginning joggers should jog for about 20 minutes per day three times per week. This does not include the time required for warming up and cooling down. Beginning joggers should ease into jogging by combining it with walking to diminish the mus-culoskeletal and cardiorespiratory stress. As fitness improves, walking time should be reduced while jogging time is increased progressively to fill the entire 20 minutes. Speed should not be increased during this time. Jogging every other day will result in enough rest between exercise sessions for the body to fully recover.

As fitness improves, walkers can exercise more often (frequency) and for a longer time (duration). Because walking is a low-impact activity, it imposes less demand than jogging upon the musculoskeletal system. The intensity of walking, however, should reflect a pace that is well tolerated and enables recovery from one work-out to the next. Reasonable exercise and health goals should be selected within these parameters. Exercisers should be patient and not attempt or expect too much too soon. Exercising beyond one's capacity will produce discomfort and pain and could pro-duce an injury— any or all of which could easily lead to discouragement, and ultimately to dropping out.

3. *Select the social contexts that are most supportive.* People can choose where and with whom they will exercise. Whether to exercise alone or with others depends upon one's preference, personality, exercise needs and goals, and compatibility with other exercisers. Evidence is available to support both approaches, and each has advantages.

Attractive features of the group approach include camaraderie, the possibility of developing productive social relationships with other group members, cooperation, competition, and reinforcement. The social support received from the group, particularly during the early weeks of a beginner's program, enhances compliance.[21]

Other people find that the individual approach to exercise is best for them. A 1-year study of older men and women showed that an individual home-based exercise program was more effective than a group program

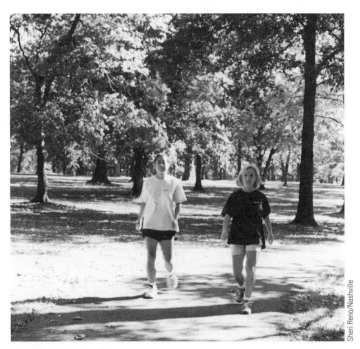

Normal gaited walking.

reinforcement. These people provide support by projecting a favorable attitude toward your exercising. A number of studies have shown that spousal support is particularly influential. Occasionally working out with a new exerciser also helps.

6. *Associate with other exercisers.* The support that others provide is more effective when they themselves are exercisers. As such, they function as role models. When people exercise together, their enthusiasm is highly visible and contagious. Walkers and joggers are eager to talk about their knowledge and experiences, and in this way participants will gain new ideas and techniques that will help to motivate them to continue their exercise program.

7. *Emphasize consistent exercise over superior performance.* Developing physical fitness and enhancing health takes time and patience. Some beneficial changes should begin to appear within the first 3 to 4 weeks. These can become a springboard for further gains.

8. *Keep a progress chart.* Keeping a daily record is helpful because this written information objectively shows the rate and amount of progress. Looking back at the record and observing the gains can be a source of motivation when a person becomes discouraged. The recording chart should reflect body weight; type, amount, and duration of exercise; and resting and exercise heart rates. (See Chapter 3 for complete discussion.) The chart should allow room for comments. Figure 2.2 provides a form for keeping track of your progress.

Weighing oneself before and after the workout is important, particularly in hot weather when fluid loss can become a major problem. Most of the weight lost during the workout is in the form of liquid, so the difference between pre- and post-exercise weight is an approximation of the amount of fluid lost. A body weight loss of 2 percent indicates slight dehydration.[23] A 3 percent loss is still

in promoting their adherence to exercise.[22] The researchers found that the group exercise program was too inconvenient over the course of the year. Convenience and accessibility of the exercise facility affected adherence to the group program. Unless these two factors are resolved satisfactorily, the independent approach might be best for that population as a whole.

4. *Exercise with a buddy.* Two people with similar training routines and compatible levels of physical fitness can provide motivational support for each other. Buddies can exchange knowledge about fitness training, nutrition, and a host of other topics of common interest to them. A bonus of the buddy system is that it becomes more difficult to skip a workout—even when the person would rather do something else—when someone is waiting at a designated time and place.

5. *Enlist the support of those who are important to you.* Friends, mates, other family members, and co-workers—people with whom you interact frequently and whose advice you value—can be important sources of motivation, encouragement, and

| DATE | BODY WEIGHT | | EXERCISE | | INTENSITY** | | | COMMENTS |
	Pre-Exercise	Post-Exercise	Type	Duration*	RHR	THR	PE	

*Time, distance, etc.
**RHR = resting heart rate; THR = training heart rate; PE = perceived exertion

Figure 2.2 Progress chart.

safe, a 5 percent loss is considered borderline, and an 8 percent loss is dangerous.[24] The loss of 1 pound of body weight is approximately equal to 1 pint of fluid loss.

Determining or approximating fluid loss is one of the functional aspects of the progress chart. Over the long term, trends in weight loss, distance covered, and heart rates (exercise and resting) will become discernible, and a record of improvement will become apparent.

9. *Exercise to music.* Music can be motivational, it provides rhythm, and it tends to take the mind off the effort associated with walking and jogging.[25] Researchers at The Ohio State University tested experienced runners with and without upbeat music.[26] The runners stated that music made the exercise bout seem easier. The researchers ran both trials, one with and one without music, at the same workload. Measures of working heart rate and blood lactate indicated that the runners were working equally hard on both trials; only their perceptions of the difficulty of the workload had changed. Music can be provided easily indoors, and portable radio headsets are popular among outdoor walkers and joggers.

A word of caution regarding the use of radio headsets: They are fine for indoor exercise or for walking or jogging on a running track. Outdoor use of headsets, however, especially when walking or jogging in areas where there is automobile, bus, and truck traffic, is distracting and intensifies the danger of their being hit.

10. *Set a definite time and place for exercise.* The exerciser should set a definite time and a convenient place during the early stages of the exercise program, resolving to walk or jog at least three times per week. The exerciser should schedule the workout just as any other important activity. Exercisers should resist temptations to replace the workout with some other pursuit that is more appealing. Skipping workouts becomes habit-forming quickly; the more you do it,

the easier it becomes. After becoming hooked on exercise (it takes 3 to 6 months), the time and place can be varied to meet changing environmental conditions (weather that is too hot, too humid, too wet, too cold, and so on), work schedules, and other conflicting responsibilities.

When is the best time of day to work out? The best time to work out is when it most conveniently fits into the daily schedule. But there are occasions when exercise should be scheduled to best meet one's goals. For instance, if stress reduction and weight loss are the goals, the best time for exercise seems to be immediately at the end of the workday and before dinner. This serves two purposes:

- It metabolizes the stress products that have accumulated in the blood during the day.

- It temporarily suppresses the appetite, resulting in the consumption of fewer calories at dinner.

If lack of time is resulting in missed workouts, the exerciser might try exercising less frequently but more intensely. Although this approach increases the potential for injury, it is better than abandoning the program completely. Exercising fewer than three times per week will not increase the fitness level but will lessen the impact of detraining. Upon returning to the normal exercise routine, the fitness level will not have deteriorated significantly.

11. *Focus on the positives.* Novice exercisers rather quickly become aware of the negatives associated with working out—among them, muscle soreness, amount of effort required, sweating, and feeling of fatigue. These factors should not act as deterrents. The exerciser should concentrate instead on accomplishments—the sense of relaxation after exercise, the increase in energy reserves, loss of body fat and gain in muscle tissue, improvement in physical appearance, better health, improved self-concept, and overall feeling of well-being.

Focusing on the positives will help keep a person motivated and excited about exercise.

12. *Don't become obsessive about exercise.* Exercise should be relaxing and recreational but not obstructive. If a person feels and acts miserable after missing a day of exercise, this is obsessive.[27] Sometimes unplanned circumstances don't allow a person to exercise on a given day. When that happens, it can be considered as one of the two days of rest included in the exercise agenda and picked up tomorrow or the next day. People should not exercise when they are ill. Missing an occasional workout will not detract from the fitness benefits already achieved. Activity can be resumed upon recovery. Later in this text you will learn about the importance of rest to an exercise program.

13. *No exercise failures.* Exercisers can achieve physical fitness and enhance and maintain their health without competing against others or the time clock. The exercise program ultimately adopted should be enjoyable and comfortable, and it should fit the exerciser's level of physical fitness. Walking and jogging do not require complex skills. And in these noncompetitive venues, there are no last-place finishes to worry about, no embarrassment with performance, and no intimidation from others.

Terms

Extrinsic reinforcement	Self-motivation
Intrinsic reinforcement	Transtheoretical model
Positive feedback	

Summary

* Only 22 percent of Americans are active enough to improve their health status, according to the Centers for Disease Control and Prevention.

* About half of new exercisers drop out during the first 6 months after starting an exercise program.

* Among the reasons that most of the "least active" Americans give for not exercising are lack of time, work conflicts, travel requirements of the job, inconvenient or inaccessible exercise site, and poor support from family members.

* Blue-collar workers, smokers, and obese people are less likely than others to begin and sustain exercise.

* External rewards are effective in the early phase of the exercise program, and internal rewards are best for maintaining exercise.

* People can take advantage of opportunities in daily life to increase energy expenditure—by mowing the lawn, washing and waxing the car, taking the stairs instead of elevators and escalators, and so on.

* The Surgeon General's report on the importance of exercise for improving health has not motivated most sedentary people to exercise.

* Only moderate levels of exercise are needed to improve health, and this can be accomplished by walking three or four times a week.

* The transtheoretical model of behavior has useful potential for motivating sedentary people to become active and maintain an exercise program.

* A moderate level of exercise is optimal; too little exercise is likely to result in failure, and too much can result in injury and burnout.

* Most people concede that exercise is good for enhancing health and improving physical appearance, but the majority of them don't participate.

* Goals for exercise should be realistic, specific, and attainable.

* Walking is a low-impact activity that imposes less demand than jogging on the musculoskeletal system.

❖ Exercising with a group has a number of advantages for some people; others prefer to exercise on their own.

❖ Exercise buddies can motivate each other and exchange knowledge regarding physical fitness.

❖ Spouses, other family members, friends, and co-workers can be important sources of motivation, encouragement, and reinforcement.

❖ Consistency in exercising is more important than superior performance.

Notes

1. Centers for Disease Control and Prevention, *Physical Activity and Health: A Report of the Surgeon General* (Atlanta: National Center for Chronic Disease Prevention and Health Promotion, 1996).

2. A. C. King and M. Kiernan, "Physical Activity Promotion: Antecedents," *ACSM's Resource Manual,* edited by J. L. Roitman (Philadelphia: Lippincott Williams and Wilkins, 2001).

3. R. Dishman and J. Sallis, "Determinants and Interventions for Physical Activity and Exercise," in *Physical Activity, Fitness, and Health*, edited by C. Bouchard et al. (Champaign, IL: Human Kinetics Publishers, 1994).

4. King and Kiernan, Note 2.

5. P. M. Ribisl and S.A. Shumaker, "Enhancing Social Support and Group Dynamics," *ACSM's Resource Manual,* edited by J. L. Roitman (Philadelphia: Lippincott Williams and Wilkins, 2001).

6. Ribisl and Shumaker, Note 4.

7. Ribisl and Shumaker, Note 4.

8. King and Kiernan, Note 2.

9. J. Annesi, "Relevant Retention Research," *Fitness Management*, 12:10 (Sept. 1996), 42–43.

10. R. K. Dishman and J. Buckworth, "Increasing Physical Activity: A Quantitative Synthesis," *Medicine and Science in Sports and Exercise*, 28 (1996), 706–719.

11. Dishman and Sallis, Note 3.

12. CDC, Note 1.

13. A. C. King and J. E. Martin, "Physical Activity Promotion: Adoption and Maintenance," *ACSM's Resource Manual*, edited by J. L. Roitman (Philadelphia: Lippincott Williams and Wilkins, 2001).

14. CDC, Note 1.

15. "How to Get Americans Active," *AAHPERD Update* (Sept./Oct. 1997).

16. M. Clements and D. Hales, "How Healthy Are We?" *Parade Magazine* (Sept. 7, 1997), 4–7.

17. "How to Get Americans Active," Note 15.

18. King and Martin, Note 7; B. A. Brehm, "Helping Clients Change," *Fitness Management*, 13:1 (Jan. 1997), 24–26.

19. King and Martin, Note 7.

20. K. H. Cooper, *Aerobics* (New York: Bantam Books, 1968).

21. CDC, Note 1.

22. King and Kiernan, Note 2.

23. T. E. Bernard, "Environmental Considerations: Heat and Cold," *ACSM's Resource Manual*, edited by J. L. Roitman (Philadelphia: Lippincott Williams and Wilkins, 2001).

24. S. K. Powers and E. T. Howley, *Exercise Physiology* (Boston: McGraw Hill, 2001).

25. E. T. Howley and B. D. Franks, *Health Fitness Instructor's Handbook* (Champaign, IL: Human Kinetics, 1997).

26. R. J. Trotter, "Maybe It's The Music" *Psychology Today*, 8:19 (May 1984).

27. D. C. Nieman, *Exercise Testing and Prescription A Health-Related Approach* (Mountain View, CA: Mayfield, 1999).

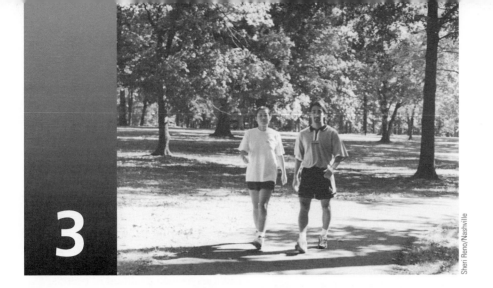

Sheri Reno/Nashville

Getting Started

Outline

If walking and jogging are to have a significant and lasting impact on our state of health, they should become lifelong activities. A sound program, based upon the guidelines and suggestions presented in this text, has the capacity to improve both the quality and the quantity of one's life. The health benefits of walking and jogging are discussed in Chapter 4. For now, we will focus on starting your program correctly, to increase the probability of success and thereby promote your adhering to exercise.

Regular and Consistent Participation

To be effective, walking, jogging, or any other form of exercise must be performed regularly. Regular participation for 2 to 3 months will yield substantial physiological and psychological benefits that ultimately might give you the motivation to continue. The major challenge for the beginning exerciser is to sustain physical activity during the early weeks of participation without losing interest or becoming injured. Enthusiastic beginners, anxious to achieve their goals rapidly, tend to overdo it in the early stage of their fitness program.

Beginners face a "catch-22" situation: They need enough motivation and enthusiasm to start and maintain the exercise habit, but too much enthusiasm can stimulate them to exercise beyond their capacity. Exercising beyond one's fitness level is not enjoyable. It is extremely uncomfortable and even potentially dangerous. If the exerciser attempts to push the program, negative feelings toward exercise will develop quickly, and soon the program, with all of its good intentions, will be discarded.

After all, how many of us are masochistic enough to endure discomfort and pain in every exercise session? Consistent participation comes about from enjoyment of exercise. Pain and enjoyment are contradictory. Therefore, novices should not become overly impatient for rapid gains. These will come soon enough.

The Medical Exam

Prior to beginning an exercise program, a medical examination is desirable for men 40 years of age and older, and for women 50 years of age and older.[1] People who are apparently healthy may participate in low- to moderate-intensity exercises without medical clearance. People at higher risk—those with two or more major risk factors—should have a medical exam that includes a physician-monitored **exercise electrocardiogram (ECG)**.

Risk factors include the coronary factors of high blood pressure, hyperlipidemias (abnormal blood fats), cigarette smoking, family history for heart disease, obesity, and a sedentary lifestyle, as well as symptoms that suggest metabolic disease (for example, diabetes, kidney disease, and liver disease). College-age adults usually can start exercising without medical clearance. Everyone should begin within their capacity and progress gradually.

Achieving Objectives

The exerciser's aims and objectives should help to determine the direction of the program and the type of physical activity selected. Weight loss, road race competition, and the development of strength are objectives that suggest different types of physical activities as well as different exercise emphases. The objective of properly conceived exercise programs should be reflected by the manner in which the principles of exercise are utilized. The extent to which each is emphasized or deemphasized is the key to accomplishing specific objectives.

Warming Up

Each exercise bout should be preceded by an 8- to 10-minute warm-up and followed by a cool-down period of equal time. Both are integral components of an exercise program. Proper warm-up and cool-down contribute to performance and the exerciser's health and safety. Sandwiched between these two components is the actual exercise program—in this text, walking and jogging.

The **warm-up** is designed to prepare the body gradually for more vigorous exercise. In approximately 10 minutes of warming up, the muscles to be involved in the activity are heated and the heart rate is allowed to increase slowly toward the rate expected during the actual workout. Rhythmic **calisthenics**, walking, slow jogging, and other low-intensity activities can be used during the warm-up to prepare the individual for exercise of greater intensity. These activities smooth the transition from inactivity to activity with minimum oxygen deprivation to the heart, muscles, and organs.

Without a proper warm-up, the heart rate would rise rapidly, forcing the body to rely upon short-term supplies of fuel to generate the energy needed for exercise. Circulation does not increase in proportion to heart rate; during a brief interval (about 2 minutes) the heart and other muscles are not fully supplied with oxygen. Early studies showed that sudden strenuous exertion without the benefit of a warm-up period produced abnormal cardiac responses that reflected oxygen deprivation, ventricular arrhythmias, and left ventricular dysfunction.[2] Later studies of healthy subjects have not confirmed the same cardiovascular abnormalities as previous studies.[3] In fact, even stable **post-myocardial** patients (heart attack patients) who had been treated with beta blocker medication did not respond abnormally to sudden exertion.[4]

At the worst, the potential for inducing a cardiovascular event during sudden physical exertion may be higher without warming up. At the least, it produces significant discomfort during the first 2 to 3 minutes after beginning exercise, and it increases the likelihood of incurring a musculoskeletal injury. This is a potentially dangerous time, particularly for those whose circulation is compromised by heart and blood vessel disease.

When the cardiorespiratory warm-up phase is complete, the muscles are stretched. At this point the walker or jogger should be sweating—indicating that the core temperature might be elevated slightly and muscle temperature is substantially elevated.[5] Both responses enhance performance and reduce the risk of physical injury. Muscles are stretched more effectively when they are heated.

The preferred method for enhancing and maintaining flexibility of the joints and elasticity of muscles and connective tissue is **static stretching**. This consists of slow, controlled movements and desired end positions that are held for 10 to 30 seconds.[6] The desired end position should

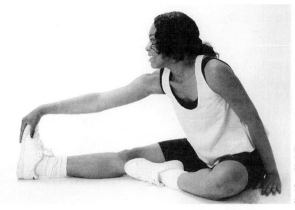

Modified hurdler's stretch. Sit with the right leg fully extended with the sole of the left foot against the inner right thigh. Keeping the right leg straight, lean forward as far as you can and attempt to reach your foot with the extended right arm. Hold 15 to 30 seconds, then switch legs and arms. This exercise stretches the hamstring muscle group in the backs of the thighs.

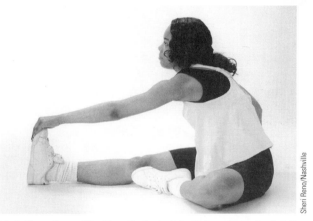

Variation of modified hurdler's stretch. This exercise is slightly more challenging than the modified hurdler's stretch in that you reach forward with the opposite hand. This will place some stretch on the lower back. Hold 15 to 30 seconds, then switch legs and arms.

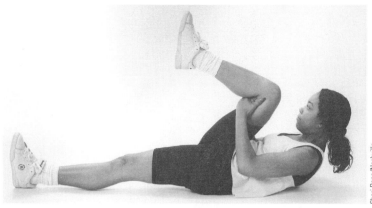

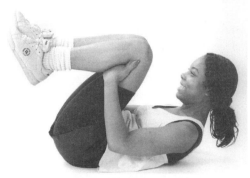

Back stretcher. To stretch the lower back, lie on your back with hands clasped at the back of the thigh of your right leg. Pull your leg to your chest and hold for 15 to 30 seconds. Switch legs.

Variation of back stretcher. From the same position as back stretcher, clasp your hands behind both thighs and pull both legs to your chest. Hold for 15 to 30 seconds.

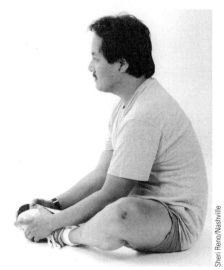

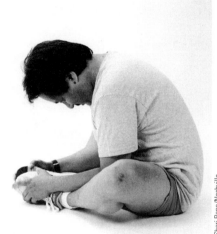

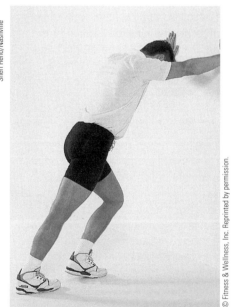

Stretching inner thighs and hips. Seated, bend your knees so the soles of the feet come together. Use your forearms to push your knees toward the floor. Hold 15 to 30 seconds.

Variation of stretching inner thighs and hips. To modify the exercise, lean forward as you push the knees to the floor. Hold 15 to 30 seconds.

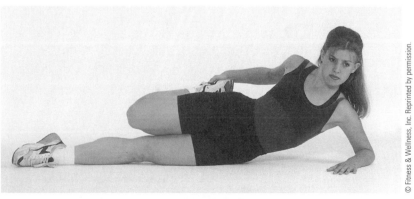

Thigh stretcher. Bend your right leg and pull that foot upward with the right hand to avoid excessive bend at the knee. Hold 15 to 30 seconds. Switch legs and hands. You may use the opposite hand to maintain balance. This exercise stretches the quadriceps muscle group at the front of the thighs.

Achilles tendon stretch. Assume a stride position with the forward leg bent at the knee and the rear leg straight with the heel planted firmly on the floor. Lean forward until you feel the stretch in the calf and achilles tendon above the heel. Hold 15 to 30 seconds. Switch legs. Be sure to point your feet straight ahead.

produce a feeling of mild discomfort but not pain. If the stretch is painful, you are stretching too forcefully and are in danger of exceeding the elastic properties of muscles. Static stretching is effective because:

- It is not likely to cause injury.
- It produces no muscle soreness.
- It helps to alleviate muscle soreness.
- It requires little energy.

Static stretches are effective and convenient, they do not require the assistance of a partner, and no equipment is necessary.

Another technique for increasing flexibility is **proprioceptive neuro-muscular facilitation (PNF).** Physical therapists have used PNF stretching for many years with patients who have neuromuscular disorders. It is more effective than static stretching in improving flexibility,[7] but it does have limitations.[8]

1. Most PNF techniques require the assistance of a partner who is competent in this system, so as not to injure the exerciser.

2. Using PNF techniques takes more time.

3. PNF is associated with more pain and muscle stiffness.

4. PNF techniques are more complex and more difficult to learn than static stretching procedures.

For these reasons, even though PNF stretching is slightly more effective than static stretching, it is not the preferred method.

Dynamic or **ballistic stretching** is not recommended because it forces muscles to pull against themselves. This type of stretching entails bouncing and bobbing movements that activate the **myotatic reflex**. Each rapid stretch sends a volley of signals from the stretch reflex to the central nervous system, which responds by ordering the stretching muscles to contract instead.

If you have dozed off while sitting in a chair, you probably have experienced the results of the stretch reflex responding to rapid stretch. Your head drops forward as you nod off, causing the neck muscles to stretch rapidly. This sudden dynamic stretch sets in motion the reflexive process that results in rapid contraction of the neck muscles and a quick return of the head to the upright position. The rapid movements in opposite directions can result in muscle soreness and possible injury.

Principles of Exercise

The six principles of exercise are intensity, frequency, duration, overload, progression, and specificity. These are discussed in turn.

Intensity

Intensity refers to the amount of energy expended per bout of exercise. For the development of physical fitness, the American College of Sports Medicine (ACSM) recommends an exercise intensity of 55/65 percent to 90 percent of maximum heart rate or 40/50 percent to 85 percent of the **cardiac reserve**.[9] Adults typically exercise at the low end of the range, whereas heart patients and healthy people with low functional capacity tend to exercise below the suggested range.[10]

The ACSM guidelines for health enhancement were issued in conjunction with the Centers for Disease Control and Prevention. According to these guidelines, a person does not have to exercise vigorously to improve health. Physical activity done at a moderate level is all that is necessary. Moderately intense physical activity consists of any activity that equals the amount of calories (energy) used to walk 3 to 4 miles per hour (mph).[11] This is a 15- to 20-minute-mile pace. When performed regularly, this activity can improve *health* by promoting weight loss and by lowering blood pressure and cholesterol levels. Exercise at this intensity, however, produces only minimum improvement in *physical fitness*. Although health can improve through moderate, regular exercise, physical activities at higher intensities produce significant improvements in *both* physical fitness and health status.

Among the several methods that can be used to determine the proper intensity for exercise are the "talk test," rate of perceived exertion (RPE), and exercise heart rate, or target heart rate.

Talk Test

The talk test is the simplest and most practical of the tests to determine intensity of exercise. If you cannot carry on a conversation fairly comfortably while walking or jogging, you might be exercising at a pace that is too intense for your level of fitness.

Rate of Perceived Exertion (RPE)

A second method involves *perception* of the effort, called **rate of perceived exertion (RPE)**. Perceived exertion is an excellent method for monitoring exercise because it produces significant indicators of effort other than heart rate. For example, it indicates overall exertional discomfort and fatigue, rate and depth of breathing, muscle fatigue, and body temperature. These

are your subjective impressions of the effort that encompasses sensory input from all of the systems associated with generation of energy for movement.

The Borg Rate of Perceived Exertion Scale (RPE) and the revised Category–Ratio RPE Scale appear in Figure 3.1. These scales provide exercisers of all fitness levels with guidelines for selecting the appropriate intensity based on their subjective perceptions of their effort. The **cardiorespiratory training effect** begins at an RPE of 12 to 13 (somewhat hard) on the original scale and 4 (somewhat strong) on the newer scale. Exercise intensities above these values will lead to the production and accumulation of lactic acid and exercise discomfort.

Lactic acid is a fatiguing metabolite resulting from the incomplete breakdown of glucose (sugar). Build-up of lactic acid in the exercising muscles produces fatigue and interferes with the muscle's ability to contract and continue to perform physical work at the same level.[12]

Values of 12 to 14 on the original RPE scale and 4 on the new scale,

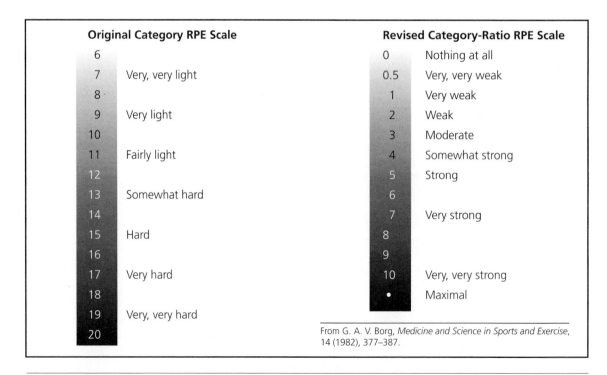

Original Category RPE Scale		Revised Category-Ratio RPE Scale	
6		0	Nothing at all
7	Very, very light	0.5	Very, very weak
8		1	Very weak
9	Very light	2	Weak
10		3	Moderate
11	Fairly light	4	Somewhat strong
12		5	Strong
13	Somewhat hard	6	
14		7	Very strong
15	Hard	8	
16		9	
17	Very hard	10	Very, very strong
18		•	Maximal
19	Very, very hard		
20			

From G. A. V. Borg, *Medicine and Science in Sports and Exercise*, 14 (1982), 377–387.

Figure 3.1 Borg's RPE scales.

approximate 40 percent to 60 percent of the **aerobic capacity**, 40 percent to 65 percent of the **heart rate reserve** (also known as cardiac reserve), and 50 percent to 75 percent of the **maximal heart rate**. The latter two concepts are explained in the following section.

Exercise Heart Rate

A third method for monitoring exercise is by **exercise heart rate** or **target heart rate (HR)**. Exercise heart rate can be determined in two ways. The first uses a percentage of the maximum heart rate, and the second uses a percentage of the heart rate reserve. The estimated maximum heart rate (HR max) must be determined as a first step for each method. This is accomplished by subtracting your age in years from the constant 220. Thus, the HR max for a 20-year-old would be:

$$\begin{array}{r} 220 \ \text{(Constant)} \\ -\ \ 20 \ \text{(Age)} \\ \hline 200 \ \text{bpm (HR max)} \end{array}$$

The HR max decreases with age, so the value for a 50-year-old would be 170 bpm (220 − 50 = 170 bpm). Regardless of age, this method is only an estimate of the HR max. The HR that the exerciser will attempt to maintain during exercise is referred to as the target HR.

Percentage of HR Max

The first method for establishing the target HR uses a percentage of the HR max. The ACSM recommends that people exercise at an intensity level somewhere between 55/65 percent and 90 percent of HR max. A person in average physical condition would select the middle of the range, or 70 percent to 80 percent of the HR max. Our 20-year-old with a HR max of 200 bpm would have a target HR of 140 bpm to 160 bpm. This is computed as follows:

$$\begin{array}{ll} 200 \ \text{bpm (HR max)} & 200 \ \text{bpm (HR max)} \\ \times .7 & \times .8 \\ \hline 140 \ \text{bpm} & 160 \ \text{bpm} \end{array}$$

People who are in better physical condition would select a higher percentage of their HR max, and those in poorer condition would select a lower percentage.

Karvonen Method

A more sophisticated approach for determining target HR is by the **Karvonen method**. This method uses the exerciser's **resting heart rate**, which is a crude measure of physical fitness, and the cardiac reserve, which is the difference between the HR max and the resting HR. Fit people in general have lower resting HRs and higher cardiac reserves than unfit people. The target for a 20-year-old in average physical condition with a resting HR of 70 bpm is calculated in the following manner using the Karvonen method:

1. Calculate HR max as before:

$$\begin{array}{r} 220 \\ -\ \ 20 \\ \hline 200 \ \text{bpm (HR max)} \end{array}$$

2. The Karvonen formula is:

THR = cardiac reserve × TI% + RHR

Where:

THR = target heart rate

Cardiac reserve = HR max − RHR

TI% = training intensity

(Get this value from Table 3.1.)

RHR = resting heart rate

Therefore:

THR = (HR max − RHR) × TI% + RHR

= (200 − 70) × .70 + 70

= 161 bpm

To use the Karvonen method, you must know your resting heart rate. According to the American College of Sports Medicine, the resting heart rate should be taken in the standing position.[13]

Learning to take HR by palpating the pulse is a skill that must be developed. The two most practical sites—and the ones used most often—are at the radial and carotid arteries. The radial pulse is palpated at the thumb

Table 3.1 Guidelines for Selecting Training Intensity Level

Fitness Level	Intensity Level (%)
Low	60
Fair	65
Average	70
Good	75
Excellent	80–90

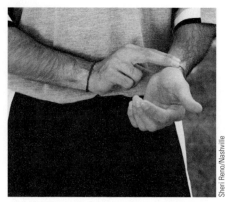

Taking the radial pulse with the fingers at the wrist.

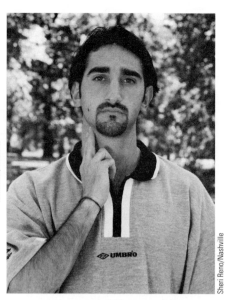

Taking the carotid pulse at the neck.

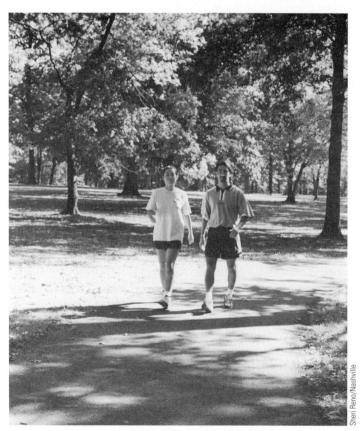

Strolling is casual walking at a pace of 3 miles per hour or slower.

side of the wrist with the hand held palm up. The carotid pulse is felt in the large artery at either side of the neck. The first two fingers of either hand are used to count the pulse rate in either location.

Because the arteries in the neck are sensitive to pressure, care should be taken when palpating the carotid pulse. Excessive pressure stretches the arteries and stimulates specialized receptors that respond reflexively by slowing the heart's rate of beating. This leads to underestimation of the actual heart rate. To circumvent this effect, the pressure applied to the carotid should not exceed the amount required to feel the pulse. To estimate the heart rate in beats per minute, count the number of pulse beats for 15 seconds and multiply that number by 4.

Frequency

Frequency refers to the number of times per week that a person participates in physical activity. To develop physical fitness, you must exercise three to five days per week at the appropriate level of intensity.[14] Fewer than three times per week is not enough of a stimulus to improve fitness, and more than 5 days per week results in diminishing returns and staleness and increases the likelihood of injury. If health improvement is the goal, however, low-intensity exercise of moderate duration (20 to 40 minutes), such as strolling (walking at 3 mph) could be done every day without resulting in orthopedic problems or staleness.

A person does not have to exercise in one continuous bout to gain benefits from it. Exercise can be split into several shorter sessions during the day. Two groups of male subjects exercised for a total of 30 minutes a day, three times per week, at 65 percent to 75 percent of their HR max.[15] One of the groups exercised continuously for 30 minutes, and the other group split the 30 minutes into three 10-minute exercise sessions. At the end of 8 weeks, the fitness level of both groups improved, but the one-exercise session group improved more. During the course of the study, however, both groups lost the same amount of weight. Short bouts of exercise spaced throughout the day is a realistic exercise option for busy people.

Days of rest are an important component of any training program. Rest is needed for physical and mental recuperation. Exercisers who don't take days off run the risk of burning out or becoming stale. There is a fine line between the amount of exercise that produces maximum gains and the amount of exercise that results in the negative effects (staleness) associated with **overtraining**. Signs of overtraining are:

1. A feeling of chronic fatigue and listlessness
2. Inability to make further fitness gains (or even a loss of fitness)
3. Sudden loss of weight
4. An increase of 5 beats or more in the resting heart rate, taken in the morning prior to getting out of bed
5. Loss of enthusiasm for working out
6. Vulnerability to injury and illness
7. Generalized anger
8. Depression.

Staleness can be psychological (lack of variety in the program or boredom after years of training) or physiological, or both. Regardless, the treatment is the same: Either stop training for a few days to a few weeks (depending upon the severity of staleness) or cut back substantially. In either case, the person should rebuild and regain fitness gradually. Prevention is the best treatment. The exerciser should recognize the signs and adjust accordingly before staleness becomes a problem.

Duration

How long a person exercises is called **duration**. In its latest guidelines, the ACSM recommended that exercise of low intensity should last a minimum of 30 minutes and be performed most days of the week.[16] This amount of exercise will improve the health status of all people and the fitness level of sedentary people. This should be considered a minimum program, though. Epidemiological data have shown that expending 1000 **kilocalories (kcals)** to 2000 kcals per week—the equivalent of walking or jogging 10 to 20 miles per week—resulted in fewer heart attacks and longer life.[17] To improve physical fitness measurably, the duration of exercise should be 20 to 60 minutes with the exercise heart rate in the appropriate zone (as determined by the Karvonen method), and the exerciser should participate 3 to 5 days per week.

There is an inverse relationship between duration (time) of exercise and its intensity during any specific workout.[18] Therefore, as the intensity of exercise increases, the duration decreases and vice versa. So walkers and joggers may expend a desired number of calories by exercising longer at a lower intensity, or they can exercise for a shorter time at higher intensities.

Overload and Progression

Overload involves subjecting the various body systems (muscular, cardiorespiratory, skeletal) to greater physical demand. **Progression** is the manner and the time in applying these demands. Periodically applying overload forces the body to adapt, and in the process it develops physical fitness. To improve, exercisers must overload on a schedule of systematic progression. After attaining the desired level of fitness, the exerciser switches from the development of fitness to the maintenance of fitness. At this point the practices of overload and progression no longer come into play.

Like other forms of exercise, overload can be applied systematically and progressively to walking and jogging. This can be accomplished by one or a combination of the following:

1. Gradually increase the distance.
2. Decrease the time you take to cover a specified distance.
3. Participate more frequently.

A good rule of thumb is to increase the frequency and duration of exercise while holding the intensity steady. After a base of fitness has been developed, intensity can be increased. Four observations might be noted regarding the application of overload:

1. Patience is necessary so as not to exercise beyond your capacity.

2. Fitness improves the most during the first 3 months of training and continues for some time, but in smaller increments.

3. Overload should be applied only when individuals are ready to accept a new challenge.

4. The 10 percent rule is necessary when applying the overload principle—that is, never increase the workload by more than 10 percent from one workout to the next.

Specificity

The body adapts according to the specific type of stress to which it is subjected—called **specificity**. The muscles, systems, and organs used in any activity adapt in the specific way they are used. Jogging does not prepare a person for swimming, nor does swimming prepare a person for cycling, because these activities are sufficiently different from each other. Jogging stresses the legs in a manner unique to that activity. The adaptations that result from jogging provide little carryover to the leg kick for swimming.

Competitors who are attempting to maximize their physical performance in a given activity are locked into a training program that is task-specific. This involves repetitive overloading of the muscles used in the event. Triathlon training provides a good example of the principle of specificity. Triathletes must train vigorously in all three events of the triathlon because no combination of training for any two of them will result in substantial improvement in the third.

People who walk or jog for health and fitness are not confined solely to these activities. They occasionally can swim, cycle, play tennis, racquetball, or other games for fun and variety. Although walking and jogging are the core of the fitness program, participants have the option of engaging in other activities on occasion if they desire.

At least 2 days of weight training are a must. Weight training should supplement walking and jogging because it stresses the total muscular system in ways that walking and jogging cannot achieve. Many people who exercise for health reasons enjoy participating in more than one physical activity. This is called **cross-training**. Still others prefer one activity because they enjoy it and it meets their needs. The point is to select an activity or activities that provide enjoyment and fulfill your health and fitness needs. Walking and jogging qualify for both.

Cooling Down After Exercise

Cooling down after exercise is just as important as warming up. Just as the body was allowed to speed up gradually, it must be allowed to slow down gradually. The body is not analogous to an auto engine that can be turned on and off with the twist of a key. Like the warm-up, cool-down should last about 8 to 10 minutes. The first phase should consist of walking or some other light activity, and the second phase should consist of the same stretching exercises that were done during the warm-up.

Phase One: Light Activity

Five minutes of continuous light activity causes rhythmical muscle contractions that prevent the pooling of blood and help to move blood back to the heart for redistribution to the vital organs. This boost to circulation after exercise is essential to the cool-down.

Inactivity during this time forces the heart to compensate for the reduced volume of blood returning to it by maintaining a high pumping rate.

The recovery period following exercise represents a potential hazard if it is not approached properly. The exerciser runs the risk of dizziness, fainting, and perhaps more serious consequences associated with diminished blood flow, the most serious of which is sudden death. Although sudden death during or immediately after exercise is rare, it does occur, and the recovery period is a likely time for its occurrence.

The worst possible cool-down procedure after fast walking or jogging is to stop all activity and stand still. The blood vessels in the legs that were dilated during exercise remain that way for a time after exercise, so blood pools in the leg veins. The downward force of gravity impedes the return of blood from the legs to the heart. Dilation of the blood vessels plus the force of gravity reduces blood flow to the heart, which limits the amount available for the body's various systems.

Because venous return of blood to the heart is reduced, the **systolic blood pressure** drops but the heart rate remains high. Systolic pressure is the pressure of the blood against the artery walls when the heart contracts. While the pressure is dropping, the hormone **norepinephrine** rises in the bloodstream. Norepinephrine constricts blood vessels and under normal circumstances raises the blood pressure.

Many authorities contend that the rise in norepinephrine after exercise is a safety mechanism in which the body reflexively attempts to maintain proper blood pressure. The stand-still posture after exercise, however, overcomes the action of norepinephrine so the pressure drops anyway. The rise in norepinephrine and drop in blood pressure coupled with a relatively high heart rate represent circulation that is out of kilter. This set of events can be a triggering mechanism for the onset of irregular heartbeats that can lead to sudden death.

The key to avoiding or at least substantially reducing the probability of sudden death after exercise is to keep moving. Walking at a moderate speed for 5 minutes will prevent blood from pooling in the legs because the contracting muscles squeeze the veins, sending more blood back to the heart. The rhythmic contractions of the leg muscles, called the "muscle pump," act as a second heart, significantly assisting it to meet the body's elevated circulatory demand. Another plus for light physical activity during cool-down is that it hastens the removal of lactic acid that has accumulated in the muscles.

Phase Two: Stretching Exercises

The second phase of cool-down calls for the same stretching exercises that were used during the warm-up. Exercisers probably will note that they tolerate stretching more comfortably after exercise, because of the increase in muscle temperature. Stretching at this time helps to prevent muscle soreness, and it provides the exerciser an opportunity to stretch the muscles that have been contracting repeatedly during the performance of exercise. This helps to maintain flexibility of the muscles and joint structures.

Bent-leg curl-ups or crunches should be added to the routine. Strong abdominal muscles are a postural aid because they provide support for the upper torso. Those who cannot do crunches correctly because of unused and weak abdominals should do modified sit-ups. Correct performance requires that the back be rounded as the participant sits up.

If you become nauseated after exercise, you should continue to walk. If you feel dizzy to the point that walking is not possible or advisable, lie down on your back. This position prevents the blood from pooling in your legs because the horizontal position nullifies the force of gravity. The feeling of nausea and subsequent vomiting when people exercise beyond their capacity is another of the body's

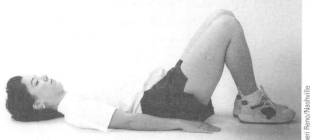

Sheri Reno/Nashville

(A) Lie on your back with knees bent and heels close to the buttocks. Extend your arms at your sides.

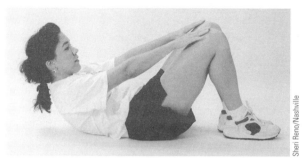

Sheri Reno/Nashville

(B) Curl up with straight arms until your fingertips contact your knees, and return to the starting position. This is a lead-up to more strenuous abdominal exercises. Start with 10 repetitions and progress from there.

Modified crunch or curl-up.

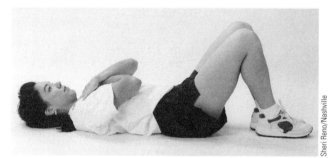

Sheri Reno/Nashville

(A) Lie on your back, knees bent, feet close to the buttocks, arms folded across the chest.

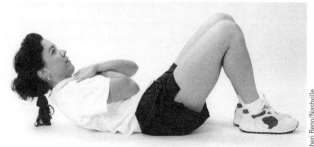

Sheri Reno/Nashville

(B) Curl up until your shoulder blades lose contact with the floor. Return to the starting position. Start with 10 repetitions and progress from there.

Crunches.

safety mechanisms. Vomiting kicks up the blood pressure toward normal, and within minutes you will begin to feel better.

The Quest for Resources

Although this text offers enough information to answer the questions of why and how to establish a walking or jogging exercise program, some people may require more help to get started. Chapter 2 presented a number of motivational strategies to help people begin and continue exercising. The first of these techniques was to develop a knowledge base for effective and safe participation in exercise.

You can begin the quest for knowledge by reading one of several reputable exercise magazines marketed to the general public. These magazines present some of the latest research information in lay terms that are easy to understand. For example, the *Fitness Management Magazine*, though oriented to health clubs, is a monthly publication written by well-qualified professional writers and exercise specialists. It covers a wide variety of aerobic and anaerobic physical activities that run the gamut from water exercises, to spinning classes, to weight training and everything in between. It is a highly informative magazine that is on the cutting edge of new trends in the exercise movement and offers many helpful hints for aspiring exercisers as well as experienced exercisers.

Walking Magazine is a monthly publication that focuses on walking as the primary mode for attaining physical fitness and enhancing health. The writers are essentially professionals who specialize in health and physical fitness. The magazine covers topics such as walking form, fitness walking, shoe selection and other walking apparel, weight control, nutrition, and other topics of interest to those who walk regularly for health and fitness.

Runner's World and *Running Times* are two monthly publications specializing in jogging and running. Professional writers and nutritionists, physicians, and exercise physiologists contribute articles to both of these magazines. Many of the articles are devoted to road racing, but the concern of many others is the dissemination of training tips for those at all levels of performance from casual joggers to serious competitors. Periodically, they evaluate jogging shoes.

With few exceptions, exercisers should include some form of resistive training in their program. Weight training is the preferred form of resistive training for many reasons. It is convenient, effective, and applicable to all ages and both sexes.

One of the best informational sources for beginners is a book entitled *Weight Training Steps to Success* by Thomas Baechle and Barney Groves. These authors are eminently qualified to write the book because, among other things, they both have earned doctorate degrees and both are certified strength and conditioning specialists through the prestigious National Strength and Conditioning Association. This book explains the selection of resistive exercises, how each contributes to strength and changes that occur in body composition, how to do each exercise, when to do each exercise, and much more. The book is accompanied by a training video that demonstrates, through slow motion, freeze frames, and illustrations, how to perform each of the exercises.[19]

The Internet is a rich source of health and physical fitness information. Refer to the appendix for web addresses where accurate and current information can be obtained.

The local library is another source of information. Reference room personnel will provide assistance in locating reputable information about health and physical fitness. While at the library, ask for information pertaining to walking and running clubs that may exist in your locale. Literally thousands of such clubs exist nationwide, most of which charge only a minimal annual fee. The benefits obtained from membership in these organizations in the form of shared information, formal information from brochures and pamphlets, camaraderie among members, and opportunities to participate in walking and running events usually make the membership fees more than worth it.

If you are fortunate enough to be employed by an organization that has a worksite fitness and health promotion program, this is a good place to initiate a physical fitness program. These programs usually are staffed by professionals who can provide many services to employees. Worksite fitness programs are growing in number with each passing year.

Community fitness centers usually are under the direction of an agency of local government. These centers charge reasonable fees and usually have a variety of fitness programs and exercise equipment as well as qualified personnel who can help clients develop effective and safe personal exercise programs.

YMCAs also offer varied programs and services at reasonable rates. Many YMCAs have upgraded their equipment, facilities, and instructional staffs in the last 10 years or so and offer opportunities to pursue fitness for beginners and experienced exercisers alike.

If membership in clubs or fitness centers is not your cup of tea and you prefer individual instruction, you might explore the possibility of hiring a personal trainer for a few weeks to a few months. Personal trainers are easy to find because most (but not all) are affiliated with fitness centers. Their fees run from 20 to 50 dollars per hour (depending upon where you live), but their expertise and one-on-one attention should get you started on the right foot. It is important to secure the services of a qualified personal trainer. To do this, investigate the trainer's background and ask the following questions:

1. Do you have a college degree in exercise science or health promotion, or one in a related field?

2. Are you certified as a Health/Fitness Instructor, Exercise Leader, Personal Trainer, or Strength and Conditioning Specialist from any of the following organizations: American College of Sports Medicine (ACSM), National Strength and Conditioning Association (NSCA), The Cooper Institute for Aerobics Research (CIAR), or the International Health, Racquet, and Sportsclub Association (IHRSA)?

3. How long have you been an exercise instructor, and what fitness organizations have you worked for previously?

If you are thinking about joining a fitness center, make sure that it:

- provides a variety of individual and group activities

- has modern aerobic and resistive exercise equipment

- has a large pool for swimming laps

- employs qualified and certified exercise instructors

- has a differentiated staff, which means that the sales force only sells memberships and the exercise instructors deal only with their clients' exercise and wellness needs.

Also, and of equal importance, are the financial costs and the arrangements to pay these costs. Do not sign a long-term contract, and do not pay for services well in advance of their receipt. Shop around for the best deal available for your needs and checkbook. Find out whether they offer family plans at a discount and provide discounts for the elderly, if applicable. Finally, before you sign any contract with a fitness club, check their rating with the Better Business Bureau.

Terms

Aerobic capacity	Norepinephrine
Ballistic stretching	Overload
Calisthenics	Overtraining
Cardiac reserve	Post-myocardial
Cardiorespiratory training effect	Progression
Cross-training	Proprioceptive neuromuscular
Duration	facilitation (PNF)
Dynamic stretching	Rate of perceived
Exercise electrocardiogram (ECG)	exertion (RPE)
Exercise heart rate	Resting heart rate
Frequency	Specificity
Heart rate reserve	Static stretching
Intensity	Systolic blood
Karvonen method	pressure
Kilocalories (kcals)	Target heart rate
Maximal heart rate	(HR)
Myotatic reflex	Warm-up

Summary

❖ Prior to starting an exercise program for men 40 years of age and older and for women 50 years of age and older, a medical exam is desirable.

❖ The exerciser's aims and objectives should help to determine how long, how hard, and how often to exercise.

❖ A warm-up prior to exercise is needed to raise muscle temperature, gently raise the heart rate, and stretch the muscles and joints.

❖ Static stretching techniques are preferred to dynamic (ballistic) stretching.

❖ PNF (proprioceptive neuromuscular facilitation) is more effective than static stretching but requires a partner, takes more time, is associated with more pain and muscle stiffness, and is more complex than other forms of stretching.

❖ Intensity refers to the amount of energy expended per bout of exercise.

❖ Intensity can be monitored by the talk test, perceived exertion, or target heart rate.

❖ For the development of fitness, the ACSM recommends an intensity level equal to 55/65 percent to 90 percent of the HR max.

❖ For the development of health, the ACSM recommends moderately intense exercise (walking 3 to 4 mph).

❖ The Karvonen method for determining target heart rate uses the resting heart rate and cardiac reserve.

❖ The most common sites for taking the pulse are the radial artery at the wrist and the carotid artery at the side of the neck.

❖ The ACSM recommends that aerobic exercise be performed three to five times per week to develop physical fitness and preferably all days of the week for improving health.

❖ Exercise that is too hard, too long, or performed too often can lead to staleness.

❖ The ACSM recommends that exercise should last a minimum of 30 minutes and be done most days of the week.

❖ The muscles, systems, and organs used in any given activity are the ones that adapt, and they do so in the specific way in which they are used.

❖ Overload is an increase in the intensity or volume of physical exercise.

❖ Progression is the systematic application of overload.

❖ Resources that can be explored for getting the exercise program "off on the right foot" include:

  ❖ reputable periodicals and magazines

  ❖ Internet

  ❖ local library

  ❖ walking or jogging club

  ❖ workplace fitness and wellness programs

  ❖ community fitness center

  ❖ YMCA fitness program

  ❖ personal trainer

Notes

1. American College of Sports Medicine, *ACSM's Guidelines for Exercise Testing and Prescription* (Philadelphia: Lippincott Williams and Wilkins, 2000).

2. R. J. Barnard et al., "Cardiovascular Responses to Sudden Strenuous Exercise—Heart Rate, Blood Pressure, and ECG," *Journal of Applied Physiology*, 34 (1973), 833; C. Foster et al, "Effects of Warm-Up on Left Ventricular Responses to Sudden Strenuous Exercise," *Journal of Applied Physiology*, 53: 380–383, 1982.

3. R. M. Chesler et al., "Cardiovascular Response to Sudden Strenuous Exercise: An Exercise Echocardiographic Study," *Medicine and Science in Sports and Exercise*, 29:10 (1997), 1299–1303.

4. R. A. Stein, H. J. Berger, and B.L. Zaret, "The Cardiac Response to Sudden Strenuous Exercise in the Post Myocardial Infarction Patient Receiving Beta Blockers," *Journal of Cardiopulmonary Rehabilitation*, 6 (1986), 336–342.

5. J. E. Kovaleski, L. R. Gurchiek, and A. W. Pearsall, "Musculoskeletal Injuries: Risks, Prevention, and Cure," *ACSM's Resource Manual*, edited by J. L. Roitman (Philadelphia: Lippincott Williams and Wilkins, 2001).

6. ACSM, "The Recommended Quantity and Quality of Exercise for Developing and Maintaining Cardiorespiratory and Muscular Fitness, and Flexibility in Healthy Adults," *Medicine and Science in Sports and Exercise*, 30:6 (1998), 975–991.

7. D. C. Nieman, *Exercise Testing and Prescription A Health-Related Approach* (Mountain View, CA: Mayfield, 1999).

8. D. M. Fredette, "Exercise Recommendations for Flexibility and Range of Motion," *ACSM's Resource Manual*, edited by J. L. Roitman (Philadelphia: Lippincott Williams and Wilkins, 2001).

9. ACSM, Note 1.

10. Nieman, Note 7.

11. R. R. Pate, "Physical Activity and Public Health," *Journal of the American Medical Association*, 273:5 (Feb. 1995), 402–407.

12. R. A. Robergs and S.O. Roberts, *Exercise Physiology for Fitness, Performance, and Health* (Boston: McGraw Hill Higher Education, 2000).

13. ACSM, Note 1.

14. ACSM, Note 6.

15. ACSM, Note 6.

16. ACSM, Note 6.

17. I-M Lee et al., "Exercise Intensity and Longevity in Men, The Harvard Alumni Study," *Journal of the American Medical Association*, 273:15 (1995), 1179–1184.

18. R. G. Holly and J. D. Shaffrath, "Cardiorespiratory Endurance," *ACSM's Resource Manual*, edited by J. L. Roitman (Philadelphia: Lippincott Williams and Wilkins, 2001).

19. T. Baechle and B. Groves, *Weight Training Steps to Success* (Champaign, IL: Human Kinetics, 1998).

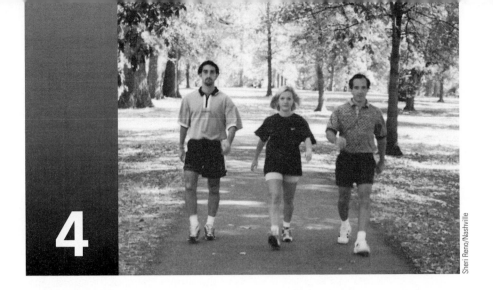

Sheri Reno/Nashville

4

Walking and Jogging for Health and Fitness

Outline

Millions of people have made the choice to walk or jog to develop aerobic fitness and enhance health. The topics of this chapter include the energy expenditure associated with both of these activities, the mechanics of walking and jogging, and tips on selecting appropriate shoes. The chapter also covers selected health benefits from regular participation in walking or jogging, and walking and jogging considerations for women, children, and elderly people.

The Fundamentals of Walking

Walking is a low-impact activity that can be done indoors or outdoors, in various climatic conditions, and on varying types of terrain. Walking first requires the proper shoes.

These Shoes Were Made for Walking

Shoes have been designed specifically for exercise walking for different terrains. Appropriate footwear adds to the enjoyment of walking and reduces the likelihood of incurring a walking-

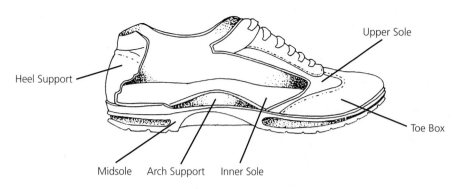

Figure 4.1 Typical walking shoe.

related injury. The following guidelines, along with the illustration in Figure 4.1, will help in selecting the proper walking shoes.

1. The shoes should be well-padded at the heel to absorb the impact of landing. Women's shoes, particularly, should be well-padded in this area because women tend to land with more force per body weight than men at all walking speeds. The heels on all walking shoes should be 1/2 to 3/4 inch higher than the sole.

2. The shoes should fit snugly at the heel and instep (the arched upper part of the foot) and should follow the foot's natural shape.

3. The outer soles should be constructed of durable solid rubber or carbon rubber for long wear. The tread should be designed for good traction.

4. The inner soles should include removable arch supports and heel cups that can be removed after a workout so they can air out and dry.

5. The upper portion of walking shoes should be constructed from leather, synthetic fabrics, or a combination. These materials allow the feet to breathe, and they provide foot comfort.

6. All walking shoes are relatively lightweight. Unless you are a competitor, you do not have to purchase the lightest shoes on the market, and actually you should not. Foot protection rather than shoe weight is most important for people who walk for health and fitness.

7. Shoes should be selected for function rather than color or fashion.

8. Beginners might do well to purchase their first couple of pairs of walking shoes from a sporting goods store that specializes in sports footwear. The professional salespeople can assist in selection and proper sizing of the shoes.

The Energy Cost of Walking

Walkers do not lose contact with the surface upon which they are traversing. A walker's advancing or striding foot lands before the rear foot leaves the ground. The rear foot supports the weight of the body while the advancing foot is swinging forward. During a brief period, both feet are in contact with the ground simultaneously. At slow speeds the normal walking gait, with its relaxed arm swing, is an efficient form of locomotion that actually conserves and reduces energy expenditure. To some extent this is a drawback to developing physical fitness, but research indicates that walking efficiency decreases and energy expenditure increases as walking speed increases.[1]

The faster you walk, the more calories you burn. This is not the case with jogging, in which speed is irrelevant. Jogging a 10-minute mile is much more comfortable, yet burns about the same number of calories as jogging a 6-minute mile.

Table 4.1 provides a comparison of the caloric expenditure for walking at different speeds for selected body weights. This table presents walking speed in miles per hour (mph), and each speed is translated into minutes and seconds to walk 1 mile at that pace. For example, walking at 3.5 mph, the walker would cover the mile distance in 17 minutes and 10 seconds (17:10). If the walker weighs 150 lbs, he or she expends 4.2 kcals/min or 72 kcals per mile ($17.17 \times 4.2 = 72$).

Table 4.1   Energy Cost of Walking, in Kcals/Minute

Body Weight (lbs.)	Walking Speed (mph)						
	2.0 (30 m/m)*	**2.5** (24 m/m)	**3.0** (20 m/m)	**3.5** (17:10 m/m)	**4.0** (15 m/m)	**4.5** (13:20 m/m)	**5.0** (112 m/m)
120	2.3	2.6	3.0	3.4	4.4	5.6	7.2
150	2.8	3.3	3.7	4.2	5.6	7.0	9.0
180	3.4	4.0	4.5	5.0	6.7	8.4	10.8
210	4.0	4.6	5.2	5.9	7.8	9.9	12.6

*m/m = minutes

Note: To find the kcals expended per minute, locate the appropriate body weight and move horizontally until you reach your speed of walking. Kcals expended per minute is located where the two intersect. For example, a 180-lb. person walking at 4 mph would expend 6.7 kcals/min. Kcals per mile would equal 100.5 (15 m/m × 6.7 = 100.5 kcals/m). If this same individual walks at 4 mph for 40 minutes, the kcals expended are 40 × 6.7 = 268 kcals.

Note that seconds must be converted into hundredths of a minute by dividing the number of seconds by 60 (10 ÷ 60 = .166). **Kilocalories,** or Kcals denote the caloric value of foods, and this designation will be used throughout the text.

Table 4.1 indicates that the kcal cost of walking increases significantly at speeds above 3.5 mph. This is primarily because we become less efficient as walking speed rises above 3.5 mph. The differences in kcals expended in walking 5 mph versus 3 mph is 34 kcals per mile for a 150-pound person. If these speeds are maintained for an hour, the difference is 318 kcals.

Body weight also has an impact on energy expenditure for both walking and jogging, as these activities are of the weight-bearing type. **Weight-bearing activities** are any sustained exercises performed against the force of gravity.[2] By way of comparison, walking and jogging are classified as weight-bearing, whereas swimming and stationary cycling are non-weight-bearing.

Transporting one's body weight from point A to point B in the upright position through muscle power requires more energy for heavier people than lighter people. Walking at 3.5 mph, a 120-pound person burns 3.4 kcals/minute, while a 210-pound person burns 5.9 kcals/minute. This is a difference of 2.5 kcals/min for every minute walked, and a 150-kcal difference for 60 minutes.

Walkers can use certain techniques to increase the aerobic challenge as well as the energy they expend per workout. The simplest way to accomplish both is to quicken the pace, but this must be done slowly, progressively, and systematically. If you have only 30 minutes to exercise, a slightly faster pace will allow you to cover more distance, it will improve your aerobic capacity, and it will burn more calories.

A second option is to use **interval training** techniques, in which the pace is alternated between your regular speed and a faster speed.[3] The faster speed should allow you to talk, but only a few breathless words at a time. You should integrate faster walking speeds systematically and slowly. In the beginning the ratio of your regular speed to the faster speed should be about three to one. For example, if you can sustain the faster pace for 1 minute, you should sustain the regular pace for 3 minutes. The cycle should be repeated until you cover the required distance or the time allotted for the workout ends. As you become more physically fit, you should increase the time spent walking faster and decrease the time spent walking slower until they eventually even out.

Studies have shown that the average preferred walking speed of healthy young adults is 3.24 miles per hour (mph), and healthy elderly people (about 70 years of age) prefer to walk at 2.9 mph.[4] Physically active people

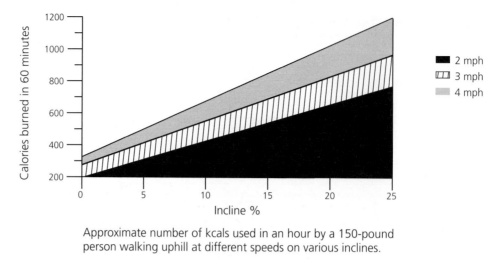

Approximate number of kcals used in an hour by a 150-pound person walking uphill at different speeds on various inclines.

Reprinted by permission from the University of California at Berkeley *Wellness Guide to Lifelong Fitness*, © Health Letter Associates, 1993. www.wellnessletter.com.

Figure 4.2 Kcals used walking uphill.

seem to prefer faster average walking speeds of 3.5 to 3.7 mph. Speeds that are measurably faster than the average for each group would constitute the faster walking intervals for each.

The energy expenditure of walking also can be increased by swinging the arms vigorously or by swinging hand-held weights. A word of caution: Vigorously swinging hand-held weights can result in shoulder soreness or injury. It also might lead to abnormally high blood pressure if the weights are gripped tightly. Vigorously swinging the arms without weight is safer, and the difference in caloric expenditure and fitness development between the two will not be significant.

Many walkers have tried ankle weights as a means of increasing the intensity of walking. These devices are not recommended, though, because they may produce injuries, primarily by distorting the walker's natural gait.

Walking up hills increases energy demand significantly and should be part of the program. Hill walking should be approached cautiously at first, attempting steeper and longer hills as fitness improves, and walking the hills at a faster pace. Hill walking places greater stress on the knees, and it is one of the causes of chondromalacia patella (this injury is explained

in Chapter 5). To reduce the likelihood of incurring this injury, you must warm up properly and use the correct form when walking hills: Lean slightly forward from the hips and shorten your stride. This should supply you with the extra power needed to negotiate the hill.

Going downhill may be tougher because it can lead to **delayed-onset muscle soreness** in the hamstring muscles (a group of muscles in the rear of the thighs). This type of muscle soreness sets in 12 to 48 hours after having completed the workout. The recommended form for downhill walking is to lean forward slightly and maintain a shorter stride with controlled steps and bent knees. Very steep hills can be traversed by crisscrossing the hill at an angle. Caloric expenditures at different grades and different speeds are given in Figure 4.2.

Another technique for increasing energy expenditure is to carry a backpack with padded shoulder straps. Start out with a light weight—soft materials such as magazines and paperback books distributed evenly in the pack. This will require a trial-and-error effort on the first few walking trips to find the correct weight. Add more weight as your fitness level improves. If you really enjoy this approach, you might consider investing in a weighted vest (which you may find more comfortable than a backpack), which allows you to increase the weight by half-pound and 1-pound increments.

Mechanics of Walking

Walking at 3 mph is considered to be casual walking or strolling. At 4 mph, walking progresses to brisk walking, or fitness walking. Walking 5 mph and faster becomes race pace. The faster one walks, the faster the arms swing. The converse is true as well: Walking speed can be increased by concentrating on swinging the arms rapidly because leg speed tends to follow arm speed. Obviously, walking at 3 mph does not require rapid arm movement, whereas walking at 5 mph does.

The purpose in this book is not to produce race walkers but, rather, to provide solid information that will encourage regular participation in health and fitness walking. Rapid speeds are not necessary to enhance health or develop fitness. Vigorous arm swinging, however, is just as important for increasing the energy requirements of walking as it is for increasing speed. Walking at a brisk 4 mph with energetic arm swinging increases the energy cost of walking.

Proper walking technique requires an erect, but not stiff, posture, in contrast to the incorrect posture of looking down at the walking surface and bending the neck. Instead, the head is erect and scans the road surface with the eyes only. Bending the neck forward to watch where you are stepping will cause you to lean forward. This position strains the lower back, upper back, and neck. It requires the static contraction of extraneous muscles and wastes energy.

The arms should be held with a 90-degree bend at the elbows. The hands should be loosely closed and relaxed. For efficiency, the arms should swing vertically and the hands should travel no higher than the earlobes. The arms are bent at 90 degrees throughout the entire swing. Increasing walking speed

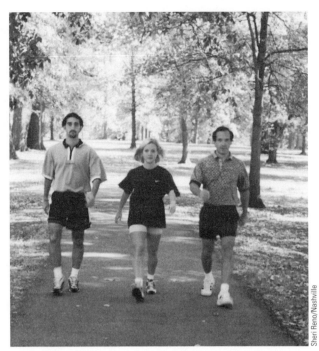

Proper walking posture is erect but relaxed.

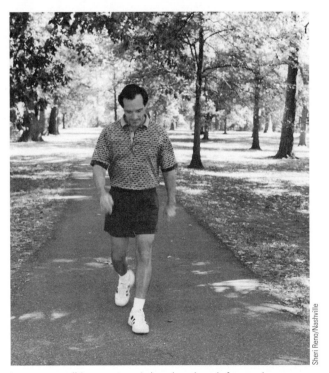

Incorrect walking posture is head and neck forward, eyes looking down.

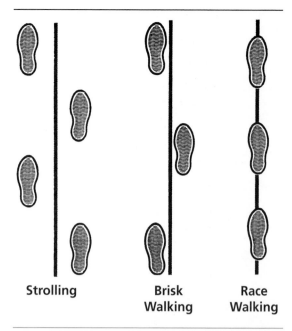

Strolling | Brisk Walking | Race Walking

Figure 4.3
Changes in foot placement at various walking speeds.

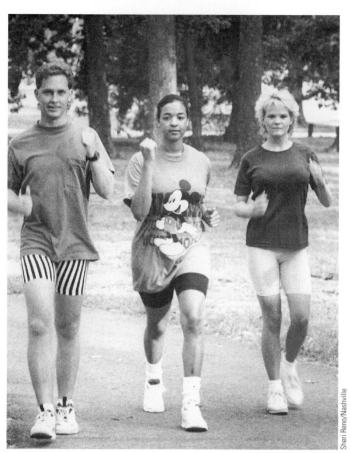

In fitness walking the arms are bent 90 degrees at the elbows and swing vigorously.

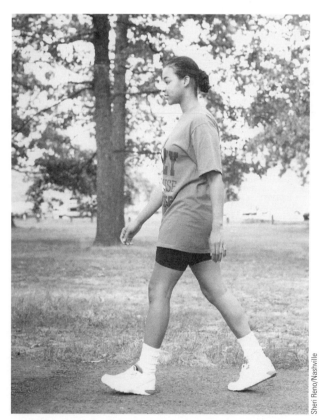

In normal-gaited walking the heel strikes first on landing, the knee is bent to take the body weight, and the push-off is from the toes of the rear foot.

is difficult if the arms swing from the shoulders in pendulum style.

In walking, the initial point of contact with the ground is the heel of the foot. This applies to all styles of walking from casual strolling to race walking. As speed increases, foot placement changes. During normal gait walking or strolling, the feet land on either side of an imaginary line that proceeds in the direction of travel, as illustrated in Figure 4.3.

As the speed increases to brisk walking, the stride lengthens and the feet land closer to the imaginary line. In race walking, the feet actually land on the line.

When the heel contacts the ground, the knee should be slightly bent. The landing foot rolls forward, accepting the weight of the body as the rear foot provides a forceful push from the toes. This is repeated rhythmically with every step.

Summary of Walking Tips

1. Beginners should walk at a comfortable pace.

2. The posture should be erect but not stiff.

3. Arms should be bent at a 90-degree angle at the elbows.

4. Hands should be loosely clenched.

5. Arm swing should be vigorous with the hands traveling no higher than the earlobes. This will increase the caloric expenditure of walking by 5 percent to 10 percent.

6. The striding leg lands on the heel and the force rolls up to the toes.

7. The rear foot provides a strong push-off.

8. The arms and legs move contra-laterally—the right arm and left leg move forward together, and the left arm and right leg move forward together.

9. The effort can be increased safely by lengthening the distance, increasing the speed, swinging the arms vigorously, and walking up hills.

10. Beginning exercisers should walk on alternate days and gradually increase the distance. When you can walk for 30 to 45 minutes without undue fatigue, you can increase the frequency to 4 or 5 days per week. If it meets your objectives, intensity can be increased after satisfying frequency and duration.

The Fundamentals of Jogging

Fitness and health objectives both can be attained expeditiously with a jogging program, and this is part of its appeal. Jogging is one of the best activities for conditioning the cardio-respiratory system, as well as most of the body's largest and most powerful muscles.

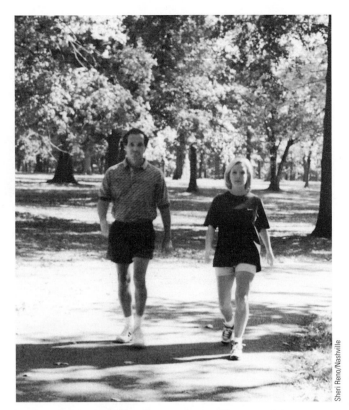

In normal-gaited walking the arms swing like a pendulum.

These Shoes Were Made for Jogging

The most important investment a prospective jogger can make is to purchase quality shoes. Proper selection is important because an appropriate, well-fitting pair of shoes can prevent or alleviate blisters, shin splints, and ankle, knee, and hip-joint injuries.

Shoes made especially for jogging have some common characteristics, shown in Figure 4.4. The heel should be about one-half inch higher than the sole, and it should be well-padded. The sole should consist of two separate layers: The outer layer should be made of a durable rubberized compound for traction and longevity, and the inner layer should be thick and pliable and made of shock-absorbing material.

The heel and sole preferably flare out so the impact with the ground can be distributed over a wider area. This is crucial because the jogger's foot hits the ground 1,500 to 1,700 times per mile and each foot strike absorbs a force equivalent to three times the

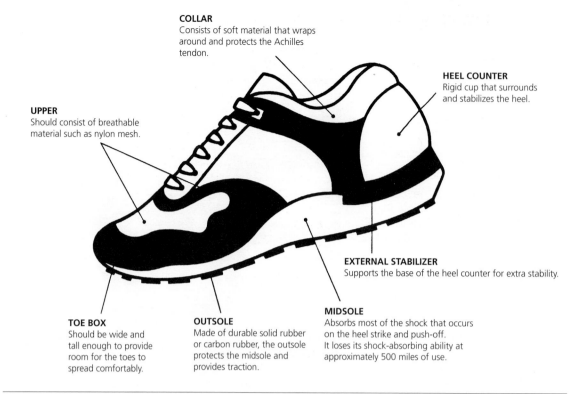

COLLAR
Consists of soft material that wraps around and protects the Achilles tendon.

HEEL COUNTER
Rigid cup that surrounds and stabilizes the heel.

UPPER
Should consist of breathable material such as nylon mesh.

EXTERNAL STABILIZER
Supports the base of the heel counter for extra stability.

TOE BOX
Should be wide and tall enough to provide room for the toes to spread comfortably.

OUTSOLE
Made of durable solid rubber or carbon rubber, the outsole protects the midsole and provides traction.

MIDSOLE
Absorbs most of the shock that occurs on the heel strike and push-off. It loses its shock-absorbing ability at approximately 500 miles of use.

Figure 4.4 Characteristics of a typical jogging shoe.

body weight.[5] It should come as no surprise that the incidence of overuse injuries rises proportionately to the number of miles jogged.

Flexibility, another characteristic of a good shoe, can be determined by grasping the heel in one hand and the toe in the other and bending it. If it does not bend easily, it is too stiff and inflexible for jogging.

Proper fit is essential. The shoes should be one-half inch longer than the longest toe, and the toe box should allow enough room for the toes to spread. The toe box should be high enough not to pinch the toes. The heel of the foot should fit snugly in the padded heel of the shoe for maximal support and minimal friction. The shoe should have a good, firm arch support.

When purchasing a pair of shoes, you should wear the same type of sock you will wear when jogging, to minimize errors in sizing. Some attention also should be given to shoe maintenance. It's best to own more than one pair of shoes so they can be rotated from workout to workout. One pair will suffice, however, if they are allowed to dry between workouts.

Shoes should be inspected periodically and discarded if they wear deep into the outer layer. As the shoe wears, the angle of the foot strike changes, producing forces at sites in the legs and hips to which the jogger is unaccustomed. This increases the likelihood of injury.

Of the shock-absorbing qualities of jogging shoes, 30 percent dissipates at about 500 miles of wear, regardless of price, brand, or type of construction.[6] At that point it is best to replace your jogging shoes.

Jogging shoes should be purchased from a store that specializes in the sale of sports footwear. The professional salespeople will suggest shoes in your price range that are appropriate to your needs. Selecting a jogging shoe can be intimidating because there are literally hundreds of models from which to choose. *Running Times* and *Runner's World* evaluate running shoes periodically. Their evaluation is probably more objective than that of a salesperson at the local running shoe store. The September 2001 edition of *Running Times* presents the results of an evaluation of 36 different models of running shoes from 17 different manufacturers.[7]

Energy Cost of Jogging

The energy cost of jogging for a given body weight is about the same regardless of speed. In fact, the net energy cost of jogging (total kcals used minus kcals that would be used while at rest) is exactly the same. Table 4.2 provides the gross and net kcals used by selected body weights at different speeds. The first line for each weight presents the gross and net kcals per minute, and the second line presents the gross and net kcals per mile.

Note that the net kcals do not change with speed, but the gross kcals change with speeds slightly for the same body weight. An individual weighing 120 pounds uses the same number of net kcals per mile whether he or she jogs at 4 mph or 8 mph. At 8 mph the individual will be generating energy at twice the rate expended at 4 mph but will be jogging for only half the time, so the net kcals expended per mile will be the same. The gross expenditure per mile actually decreases as speed increases, but the reduction is insignificant. Joggers can shorten the workout by running faster and still use the same number of kcals per mile, or they can jog slower at a more comfortable rate of speed for a longer time and expend about the same number of total kcals.

The net caloric cost of jogging 1 mile is twice that of walking a mile on level ground at moderate speeds.[8] But at higher rates of walking speed (5 mph or faster), the caloric cost of running 1 mile is only 10 percent more than walking 1 mile (see Table 4.3). Notice that the net energy expenditure for walking is quite stable up to 3.5 mph. Above this speed, the net kcals increase rapidly so the energy expenditure for walking and jogging come closer together. A 150-pound person walking and jogging at the same speed expends similar amounts of energy on a per-mile basis.

For example, if this 150-pound person walks and jogs at 5 mph, the difference in energy expended per mile is only 10 kcal. Examine Tables 4.2 and 4.3 closely, and compare the two for kcal burned for different body weights and different speeds. Based upon your exercise objectives, the data in these tables might contribute to your selecting the exercise mode that is right for you.

Table 4.2 Gross/Net Kcal Expenditure for Jogging*

Body Weight (lbs.)	MPH Speed (min per mile)	4.0 15.0	5.0 12.0	6.0 10.0	7.0 8.30	8.0 7.30	9.0 6.40	10.0 6.0
120	Kcals (min)	6.5/5.5	7.8/6.9	9.2/8.3	10.8/9.8	12/11.1	13.3/12.4	14.8/13.8
	Kcals (mile)	97/83	94/83	92/83	92/83	90/83	89/83	89/83
150	Kcals (min)	8.1/6.9	9.8/8.7	11.5/10.4	13.4/12.2	15.1/13.9	16.8/15.6	18.5/17.3
	Kcals (mile)	121/104	118/104	115/105	114/104	113/104	112/104	111/104
180	Kcals (min)	9.7/8.3	11.8/10.4	13.8/12.5	16.1/14.7	18.1/16.7	20.1/18.7	22.2/20.8
	Kcals (mile)	146/125	141/125	138/125	137/125	136/125	134/125	133/125
210	Kcals (min)	11.3/9.7	13.8/12.2	16.1/14.6	18.8/17.2	21.1/19.5	23.4/21.9	25.8/24.3
	Kcals (mile)	170/146	165/146	161/146	160/146	158/146	156/146	155/146

* The first number in each set is gross kcals; the second number is net kcals. The first set of numbers for each body weight is kcals per minute for each speed; the second set is kcals per mile for each speed. Example: A 150-lb person jogging at 6 mph will expend 11.5 gross kcals/min; 10.4 net kcals/min; 115 gross kcals/mile; 105 net kcals/mile.

Table 4.3 Gross/Net Kcal Expenditure for Walking*

Body Weight (lbs.)	MPH Speed (min per mile)	2.0 30	2.5 24	3.0 20	3.5 17:8	4.0 15	4.5 13:20	5.0 12
120	kcals (min)	2.3/1.4	2.6/1.8	3.0/2.1	3.3/2.5	4.4/3.5	5.6/4.7	7.2/6.3
	kcals (mile)	69/42	63/42	59/42	57/42	66/52	75/63	86/75
150	kcals (min)	2.9/1.7	3.3/2.2	3.7/2.6	4.2/3.0	5.5/4.3	7.0/5.9	9.0/7.8
	kcals (mile)	87/52	79/52	74/52	72/52	82/65	93/78	108/94
180	kcals (min)	3.5/2.1	4.0/2.6	4.5/3.2	5.0/3.7	6.6/5.2	8.4/7.1	10.8/9.4
	kcals (mile)	104/63	95/63	89/63	86/63	99/78	112/94	129/113
210	kcals (min)	4.0/2.4	4.6/3.0	5.2/3.7	5.8/4.3	7.7/6.1	9.8/8.3	12.6/11.0
	kcals (mile)	121/173	111/173	104/73	100/73	115/92	131/110	151/132

* The first number in each set is gross kcals; the second number is net kcals. The first set of numbers for each body weight is kcals per minute for each speed; the second set is kcals per mile for each speed. Example: A 150-lb person walking at 3.5 mph will expend 4.2 gross kcals/min; 3.0 net kcals/min; 72 gross kcals/mile; 52 net kcals/mile.

Mechanics of Jogging

A comfortable erect posture with the head level encourages the correct body alignment for jogging. You should survey the path in front of you for obstacles and irregular terrain, but your neck should not be bent forward. Do not look directly in front of your feet, because this detracts from jogging efficiency and leads to muscle strain in the neck and lower back if you maintain this posture for some time.

The hands, which are loosely closed, should be carried slightly lower than the elbows for energy conservation and comfort. This posture tends to relax the neck and shoulders. The low hand position works against generation of powerful pumping action from the arms, but this is not necessary for jogging. Sprinters require power from the arm swing; joggers swing the arms for rhythm and balance. The arms should swing backward and forward and should not cross in front of the body.

The jogging stride should be short and compact, with the foot landing beneath the knee. This aids in keeping the body erect and prevents overstriding. The jogger should land softly on the heel and rock up through the ball of the foot to the toes for the push-off. The body weight transfers from the heel along the outside edge of the foot to the toes. This distributes the impact over a greater surface area and

for a longer time, resulting in smooth, energy-efficient locomotion. The landing should be essentially noiseless.

The main difference between walking and jogging is that the body is airborne during each stride while jogging. The airborne or "float" phase accounts for about 30 percent of the length of stride. The airborne phase represents one of the primary reasons the energy cost of jogging is higher than walking: More energy is required to propel the body into the air with each stride. Overstriding is to be avoided. When the ankle is forward of the knee upon landing, the foot acts as a brake to forward motion. This reduces the efficiency of jogging and also puts stress upon the knee joint, increasing the probability of injury.

Mechanical factors that make jogging such a good aerobic conditioner are the very ones that can produce injury. The fact that joggers are airborne with every step results in a high-impact landing. The ground reaction force when the foot strikes the surface, coupled with the subsequent push-off that propels the body upward, is approximately equal to three times the body weight. Because the average jogger steps between 1,500 and 1,700 strides per mile, the knees, hips, and feet absorb the shock of landing that many times. Multiply these values by the number of miles covered in a week, and you can understand the cumulative forces operating on the jogger.

But joggers make a number of biomechanical adjustments that help to dissipate the shock. For example, the flexed position of the knee and ankle when the heel strikes the ground allows the contracting muscles to stabilize the involved joints. In the contracted position the muscles act as shock absorbers that diffuse the impact of landing. By the time the shock reaches the hip joint, it has been effectively reduced to one-sixth of its original intensity. These adjustments allow joggers to run for many years without serious injuries or premature wear of the joints.

Despite this remarkable adaptability, most joggers sustain an injury or two at some time during their many years of jogging. Fortunately, most of these injuries are minor and respond well to rest or treatment.

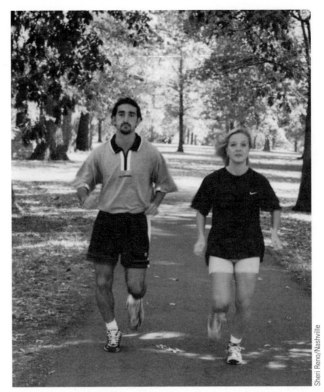
Correct jogging form requires an erect but relaxed posture.

Summary of Jogging Tips

1. Sedentary people should ease into jogging, beginning by walking and progressing to a combination of walking and jogging. In the beginning, much more time is spent walking. As fitness improves, walking time is reduced and jogging time is increased until eventually the person will be able to jog for the entire exercise session.

2. The intensity (pace) should be at a low level at first. Frequency and duration should be increased before increasing the intensity.

3. Jogging posture features an erect, but not stiff, body position, with the head level and eyes moving to scan the road ahead.

4. The hands should be slightly lower than the elbows during the arm swing because this promotes relaxation of the neck, shoulders, and jaw.

5. The arms should not swing across the body because this results in rotational sway that decreases efficiency.

6. The correct form is to land on the heel so the large muscles of the legs will absorb the shock of landing.

7. A quality pair of jogging shoes is a must, particularly for running on city streets and sidewalks.

Health Benefits of Walking and Jogging

During the last three to four decades, literally hundreds of studies have been completed and reported in professional journals regarding the relationship between exercise and health. The mainstream print and electronic media have carried many stories about the physical fitness movement. Dozens of Internet sites deal with physical fitness and health. As a result, locating information about exercise and the benefits of the physically active life is relatively easy. Still, more than 60 percent of Americans continue to remain either physically inactive or are not active enough to positively affect their health.[9]

Only about 23 percent of adults participate in regular, vigorous physical activity that involves large muscle groups in dynamic movement for at least 20 minutes, three or more days per week.[10] Another 15 percent of U.S. adults report physical activity of any intensity five or more days per week for at least 30 minutes per workout. An alarming 40 percent of U.S. adults do not participate in any regular physical activity. Yet, virtually all Americans believe that regular participation in physical exercise is one of the best prescriptions for a long and healthy life, although most would be hard-pressed to articulate why that is so.[11]

The major health benefits derived from consistent participation in walking, jogging, or any other aerobic activity are described below. Furthermore, the evidence clearly shows that moderate-intensity exercise produces all or most of the health benefits that are associated with higher-intensity exercise.

To begin with, many long-term studies have shown that physically active people generally outlive their physically inactive counterparts.[12] Of tremendous importance is that active elderly people maintain their functional independence into old age. The end result is an increase in the quality as well as the quantity of life.[13]

Coronary heart disease is the leading cause of death and disability in the United States. Physically active people have about half the risk of developing coronary heart disease as those who are physically inactive.[14] A sedentary lifestyle contributes to 250,000 deaths annually in the United States, mostly from heart disease or medical problems such as diabetes, hypertension, and obesity, all of which substantially raise the risk for heart disease.[15] Not only does exercise protect those who do not have heart disease, but it also reduces the risk in people with established heart disease by about 25 percent.

Thirty minutes of moderate to vigorous walking or jogging reduces the risk for **strokes (brain attacks)** in females.[16] Similar data are not yet available for males, but the best guess is that they would respond in a similar fashion.

The two major lifestyle risk factors for developing **Type II diabetes** are overweight and lack of physical activity. Both of these lifestyle conditions increase cellular resistance to insulin, which is a hormone needed to transport sugar (glucose) from the blood to the cells, where it can be used to fuel cellular functions. Aerobic exercises, which have an insulin-like effect, coupled with weight loss, markedly decrease cellular resistance to insulin and may normalize the body's ability to use sugar as a fuel.[17] Brisk walking or slow jogging on a regular basis decreases cellular resistance to insulin in amounts approximately equal to more intense exercise bouts.[18]

Mild to moderately intense aerobic physical activities seem to be somewhat more effective in lowering and controlling blood pressure than are high-intensity exercises.[19] A 30-minute walk five days or more per week is all that is necessary to achieve this healthy result.

Walking and jogging are weight-bearing physical activities that increase bone density and consequently decrease the risk of developing **osteoporosis** (fragile bones that are easily broken).[20] They also improve strength of the muscles, tendons, and ligaments, thereby promoting joint stability and reducing the likelihood of injury.

Substantial data indicate that exercise (both aerobic and resistive training) should be an integral part of a weight loss program.[21] The two major roles of exercise in weight management are to prevent weight gain and to maintain weight loss after the diet ends. In addition, exercise may contribute to weight loss and health enhancement by: (a) burning calories; (b) suppressing the appetite in some people; (c) counteracting the ill effects associated with obesity, such as high blood pressure, elevated cholesterol, glucose intolerance, and the like; (d) producing healthy mood changes; and (e) coping with stress.

Walking and jogging have been credited with protecting the brain as well as the heart. The mechanisms probably involve the effect of exercise on lowering blood pressure and cholesterol. Exercise also has a vasodilating effect on the arteries of the body including those that supply the brain.[22]

Walking and jogging positively affect mood states. The psychological and emotional benefits include improvement in mood, self-esteem, and self-efficacy.[23] A growing body of evidence indicates that mild to moderate depression can be improved substantially with consistent aerobic exercise. Finally, some evidence indicates that leisure-time aerobic activities and a high level of physical fitness reduce the risk of developing some forms of cancer.[24]

This summary of the health benefits of walking, jogging, and other types of exercise is just the tip of the iceberg. If we could take just the benefits listed here and press them into a pill, few Americans would refuse to buy. The problem plaguing the majority of Americans is their refusal to commit the time and effort to achieve those benefits, and as of this time there is no exercise pill.

Walking and Jogging for Special Populations

Special concerns apply to women, including pregnant women, as well as elderly people and children.

Special Concerns of Women

Although males and females are physiologically similar in some ways, they have enough differences to affect physical performance. For example, the aerobic capacity of the average female is approximately 20 percent lower than that of the average male. The difference results from the following:

1. A smaller heart size per unit of body mass

2. Lower oxygen-carrying capacity because of 10 percent to 15 percent less hemoglobin (the oxygen-carrying component of red blood cells)

3. Less muscle mass to supply the power to move their body weight

4. More inactive fat tissue to move about.

Because of their larger muscle mass, the average male is about 30 percent to 40 percent stronger than the average female. Strength is highly and positively correlated with physical performance.

Menstruation represents a significant difference between males and females. The response to menstruation among females is variable. Some women feel no different than usual, and others may experience abdominal and leg cramping, low-back pain, and mood swings. The female response to menstruation may affect physical performance markedly.

Despite the physiological differences between males and females, the responses to aerobic training are remarkably similar. On a percentage basis, the ability to deliver and extract oxygen is essentially the same in men and women. So too, are benefits such as fat loss, decreased heart rate, and increases in bone density. In addition, exercise training reduces many of the risk factors associated with the chronic diseases that are the leading causes of death in the United States. In summary, regular exercise is as important a lifestyle behavior for women as it is for men.

Exercise During Pregnancy

Women can profit substantially from exercise during pregnancy. But exercise during pregnancy should be discussed with a woman's physician. If she was actively engaged in exercise prior to pregnancy, she most likely will be allowed to continue. If she was not physically active and wishes to become active during pregnancy, she would be wise to discuss the risks and benefits with her physician. If medical

Table 4.4   Benefits of Regular Exercise for Pregnant Women

1. Improved aerobic and musculoskeletal fitness
2. Greater energy reserve
3. Reduced lower back pain during pregnancy
4. Faster recovery from labor
5. Shortened period of labor with less pain
6. Improvement in psychologic well-being
7. Less likely to encounter postpartum depression
8. Helps to establish exercise as a lifestyle behavior
9. Quicker return to prepregnancy weight and fitness level
10. Less weight gain during pregnancy

Adapted from ACSM, *ACSM's Guidelines for Exercise Testing and Prescription.*
Philadelphia: Lippincott Williams and Wilkins, 2000.

clearance is granted, she should be directed to a trained exercise specialist who is qualified to prescribe exercise during pregnancy. The health and fitness benefits of aerobic exercises during pregnancy are listed in Table 4.4.

The American College of Obstetricians and Gynecologists (ACOG) has developed the following guidelines for exercise during pregnancy.[25] Pregnant women should:

1. Engage in aerobic exercise—walking is most often recommended—three times per week.

2. Reduce the intensity of exercise as pregnancy progresses, and then shift from higher-impact weight-bearing activities such as jogging to lower-impact activities such as walking, and then non-weight-bearing activities such as swimming and stationary cycling.

3. Avoid activities that place a high reliance on balance.

4. Avoid exercises performed while lying on the back after the third month of pregnancy. This position encourages a shift in blood supply away from the uterus, which has potential, although unproven, consequences for the fetus.

5. Avoid prolonged motionless standing.

6. Avoid activities that significantly raise the core maternal body temperature.

7. Be careful not to dehydrate while exercising.

Breast Support During Exercise

All women, regardless of breast size, would be well-served to invest in a quality sports bra because it contributes to comfort by limiting breast movement. In addition to providing support, a quality sports bra has wide straps that won't slip off the shoulders, has a wide band at the bottom to reduce the likelihood of riding up, is made of nonabrasive material, and is seamless to avoid chafing.

Exercise and the Elderly

People over 65 years of age represent the fastest growing group in the United States.[26] This is attributable to many factors including advances in medicine and medical care of the elderly, as well as their adopting lifestyle behaviors conducive to longer life.

The year 2000 census indicated that there were more than 51,000 centenarians (people 100 years old and older) and that more than 1,400 were super-centenarians (age 110 years or older). Notwithstanding this laudable achievement, the reality is that the elderly require more medical care than any other age group. On average, the last few years of their lives are characterized by a medicated existence, usually to combat more than one chronic disease. This presents an enormous challenge to the health care system and at the same time affords a great opportunity to educate all Americans about the importance of practicing lifestyle behaviors that have the potential to prevent or delay diseases that become prominent later in life.

Studies have shown that physicians have the greatest influence on changing the behaviors of the general public.[27] But physicians are busy with their major responsibilities—diagnosing and treating illness, as well as staying abreast of the rapidly occurring innovations in medicine. This is what they are trained to do. Education takes time and at this point is secondary to diagnosis and treatment, but physicians should recognize that it would be time well spent, as they have considerable influence over patients' behavior. Before this occurs on a national scale, the medical community will have to adopt a different mindset.

So much evidence has accrued showing that the elderly benefit from exercise in much the same way as young people that it has become an article of faith (see Table 4.5). The elderly do need to be more cautious in their selection of activities and in their level of exercise intensity. And it goes without saying that the elderly should obtain medical clearance before embarking on an exercise program. Because exercise reduces the risk of developing most chronic diseases, and because the elderly are the main victims, it makes good sense for them to become more active. Although establishing the exercise habit early in life is best, it is never too late to start.

Walking is an excellent exercise for the elderly. As a low-impact activity, it carries a low risk, and it can be done almost anywhere, anytime, alone or with others, and all it costs is a good pair of walking shoes. Surveys show that it is the favorite type of exercise for elderly people, and it is the activity they are most likely to sustain. Walking five or six days per week should be supplemented with a light-to-moderate weight-training program.

The Need for Children to Exercise

Children have a natural inclination to play, but today there is heavy competition from inactive pursuits. Television viewing, video games, movies, and computers are cutting into active playtime for children and adolescents. One of the unhealthy results of choosing inactive play over active play is the increasing number of overweight or obese youngsters. In 1999 an estimated 13 percent of children aged 6 to 11 and 14 percent of adolescents ages 12 to 19 were overweight. This represented a 2 percent to 3 percent increase between 1994 and 1999.[28]

Table 4.5 Health Benefits of Regular Exercise for the Elderly

Lowers	Helps
1. the risk of dying prematurely especially from heart disease	1. reduce high blood pressure in people who already have it
2. the risk of developing diabetes	2. control body weight
3. the risk of developing high blood pressure	3. build and maintain healthy bones, muscles, and joints
4. the risk of developing colon cancer	4. improve cardiorespiratory endurance and muscular strength
5. feelings of depression and anxiety	5. control swelling and joint pain associated with arthritis
6. the risk of falling and bone fractures	

Adapted from *Physical Activity and Health: A Report of the Surgeon General,* Atlanta: National Center for Chronic Disease Prevention and Health Promotion, 1996.

The percentage of overweight children nearly doubled between 1980 and 1994, and the upward trend is showing no signs of slowing down or reversing. Overweight and obesity, particularly during adolescence, tends to track into adulthood so that today's overweight youngsters will become tomorrow's overweight adults with all of the attendant risk factors.

The Surgeon General's report in 1996 estimated that half of America's youth were not physically active enough to improve cardiorespiratory fitness. This is not attributable entirely to the popularity of inactive pursuits. Another factor is the reduction of physical education programs in the public schools, many of which have been eliminated because of budgetary constraints. The loss of these programs has reduced the opportunity for youngsters to receive instruction in sport skills, as well as the opportunity to participate in vigorous physical activity. On top of that, many existing physical education programs have done little to promote lifetime physical fitness.

Parents can be effective role models of the physically active life. First, they can become exercise participants themselves, and second, they should participate in physical activities with their children on a regular basis. Family activities for fun and fitness might help to establish the exercise habit in children.

An Uncomplicated Walking Program for the Obese

Obese people tend to avoid exercise because they may be embarrassed by their appearance, or they may be poorly skilled, or they may fail to exercise for some other reason. When activities are chosen wisely, skill proficiency becomes incidental. Walking is one of the activities of choice unless an individual is excessively obese or has severe arthritis in the lower limbs. Walking is our natural form of locomotion, and it is a weight-bearing exercise. Because it is weight-bearing, it is a calorie burner for the obese because of the extra pounds that they are carrying.

The American College of Sports Medicine and the National Institute of Health recommend a walking program that has no complex guidelines and that almost anyone, obese or not, can benefit from. In addition to a good pair of walking shoes, the only requirement is a pedometer. Pedometers are small, lightweight instruments, worn on a belt or waistband, that measure the number of steps one walks (and some of them measure the number of miles as well). The person wears the pedometer every day during the waking hours. The program objective is to progress to a total of 10,000 walking steps per day.[29]

Why count steps rather than miles? Success and progress are measured in much smaller increments when steps rather than miles are counted; therefore, improvement is easier to discern. As the number of walking steps increases over time, the satisfaction that accompanies progress should motivate people to continue toward the goal of 10,000 steps. Why 10,000 steps?

It takes approximately 2,000 steps to walk 1 mile, so 10,000 steps is approximately 5 miles. Sedentary people walk an average of 2,000 to 4,000 steps in a normal day. Moderately active people average 5,000 to 7,000 steps in a normal day. A daily 10,000 steps is a worthy goal that will improve health—and all of this for the price of a pedometer (about 27 to 30 dollars) and a little effort.

Terms

Coronary heart disease	Osteoporosis
Delayed-onset muscle soreness	Strokes (brain attacks)
Interval training	Type II diabetes
Kilocalories	Weight-bearing activities

Summary

❖ Walking is a low-impact activity because both feet don't leave the ground simultaneously.

❖ Walking contributes to physical fitness and health.

❖ Walking shoes should contain certain features to make walking more enjoyable and safer.

❖ Walking is an efficient form of locomotion except at the higher speeds. The faster one walks, the more calories one burns.

❖ The energy expenditure of walking can be increased safely by swinging the arms vigorously and by walking up hills.

❖ Shoes designed for jogging are a must because they are constructed to help dissipate the forces generated on impact with the ground.

❖ The energy cost of jogging for a given body weight is about the same regardless of speed.

❖ The net caloric cost of jogging 1 mile is twice that of walking 1 mile on level ground at moderate speeds.

❖ Overstriding occurs when the ankle is forward of the knee upon landing. This should be avoided because the foot acts as a brake and stresses the knee joint.

❖ Joggers step between 1,500 and 1,700 times per mile.

❖ 60 percent of Americans are either physically inactive or not active enough to positively affect their health.

❖ Only 23 percent of U. S. adults participate in regular, vigorous physical activity.

❖ 40 percent of U. S. adults do not participate in any regular physical activity.

❖ Regular aerobic exercises contribute to longevity.

❖ Physically active people have about half the risk of developing coronary heart disease as those who are physically inactive.

❖ A sedentary lifestyle contributes to 250,000 deaths annually.

❖ Thirty minutes of moderate to vigorous walking or jogging reduces the risk for strokes.

❖ Regular walking or jogging reduces the risk of Type II diabetes.

❖ Mild- to moderate-intensity aerobic physical activity is effective in lowering high blood pressure.

❖ Walking and jogging contribute to greater bone density.

❖ Walking and jogging contribute to weight loss and weight control.

❖ Walking and jogging positively effect mood and self-esteem.

❖ Aerobic activities reduce the risk of some forms of cancer.

❖ Males and females respond to training in similar ways, with a few caveats.

❖ Exercise is beneficial during pregnancy, following guidelines developed by the American College of Obstetricians and Gynecologists.

❖ Active women should wear a good sports bra.

❖ Exercise is necessary and beneficial for elderly people, children, and people who are overweight and obese.

Notes

1. E. T. Howley and B. D. Franks, *Health Fitness Instructor's Handbook* (Champaign, IL: Human Kinetics, 1997).

2. "Ever Wonder What Counts as Weight Bearing Exercise?" *University of California Wellness Letter,* 17:8 (May 2001), 8.

3. S. Camelio, "How to Walk Off Weight," *Natural Health Magazine,* 31:6 (Aug. 2001), 70–73.

4. M. D. Grabiner and P. E. Martin, "Biomechanics and Physiology of Posture and Gait," *ACSM Resource Manual,* edited by J. L. Roitman (Philadelphia: Lippincott Williams and Wilkins, 2001).

5. W. E. Prentice, *Fitness and Wellness for Life* (Boston: WCB McGraw-Hill, 1999).

6. T. P White, *The Wellness Guide to Lifelong Fitness* (Rebus, NY: Random House, 1993).

7. Running Times Editorial Staff, "Fast Fall Shoes" *Running Times,* 289 (Sept. 2001), 1832.

8. ACSM, *ACSM Guidelines for Exercise Testing and Prescription* (Philadelphia: Lippincott Williams and Wilkins, 2000).

9. U. S. Dept of Health and Human Services, *Physical Activity and Health: A Report of the Surgeon General* (Atlanta: Centers for Disease Control and Prevention, National Center for Chronic Disease Prevention and Health Promotions, 1996).

10. C. G. Spain and B. D. Franks, "Healthy People 2010: Physical Activity and Fitness," *President's Council on Physical Fitness and Sports* (Washington, DC: President's Council on Physical Fitness and Sports, 2001).

11. Editors of the Johns Hopkins Medical Letter, "Tapping Into the 'Real' Fountain of Youth," *Health After 50,* 13:6 (Aug. 2001), 45

12. U. M. Kujala, J. Kaprio, S. Sarna, et al., "Relationship of Leisure-Time Physical Activity and Mortality: The Finnish Twin Cohort," *Journal of the American Medical Association,* 279:6 (1998), 440–444; R. S. Paffenbarger, R. R. Hyde, A. L. Wing, et al., "The Association of Changes in Physical-Activity Level and Other Lifestyle Characteristics with Mortality Among Men," *New England Journal of Medicine,* 328:8 (1993), 538–545; S. E. Sherman, R. B. D'Agostino, J. L. Cobb, et al., "Physical Activity and Mortality in Women in the Framingham Heart Study, *American Heart Journal,* 128:5 (1994), 879–884; G. A. Kaplan, W. J. Strawbridge, R. D. Cohen, et al., "Natural History of Leisure-Time Physical Activity and Its Correlates: Association with Mortality for All Causes and Cardiovascular Disease Over 28 Years," *American Journal of Epidemiology,* 144:8 (1996), 793–797; L. H. Kushi, R. M. Fee, A. R. Folson, et al., "Physical Activity and Mortality in Postmenopausal Women," *Journal of the American Medical Association,* 277 (1997), 1287–1292.

13. D. M. Buchner, "Preserving Mobility in Older Adults," *Western Journal of*

Medicine, 167:4 (1997), 258–264; B. S. Tseng, D. R. Marsh, M. T. Hamilton, et al., "Strength and Aerobic Training Attenuate Muscle Wasting and Improve Resistance to the Development of Disability with Aging," *Journal of Gerontology,* 50A (1995), 113–119.

14. Spain and Franks, Note 10.

15. Editors of Johns Hopkins Medical Letter, Note 11.

16. Editors of Johns Hopkins Medical Letter, Note 11.

17. B. N. Campaigne, "Exercise and Diabetes Mellitus," *ACSM Resource Manual,* edited by L. L. Roitman (Philadelphia: Lippincott Williams and Wilkins, 2001).

18. F. B. Hu, et al., "Walking Compared with Vigorous Physical Activity and Risk of Type II Diabetes in Women: A Prospective Study," *Journal of the American Medical Association,* 282 (1999), 1433–1437.

19. S. J. Kerry, "Exercise and Hypertension," *ACSM Resource Manual,* edited by J. L. Roitman (Philadelphia: Lippincott Williams and Wilkins, 2001).

20. J. M. Shaw, K. A. Witzke, and K. M. Winters, "Exercise for Skeletal Health and Osteoporosis Prevention," *ACSM Resource Manual,* edited by J. L. Roitman (Philadelphia: Lippincott Williams and Wilkins, 2001).

21. C. M. Grilo and K. D. Brownell, "Interventions for Weight Management," *ACSM Resource Manual,* edited by J. L. Roitman (Philadelphia: Lippincott Williams and Wilkins, 2001).

22. Editors of Harvard Medical School, "Exercise and the Endothelium," *Harvard Heart Letter,* 11:5 (Jan. 2001), 1–2,

23. Editors of Johns Hopkins Medical Letter, Note 11.

24. M. H. Whaley and L. A. Kaminsky, "Epidemiology of Physical Activity, Physical Fitness, and Selected Chronic Diseases," *ACSM Resource Manual,* edited by J. L. Roitman (Philadelphia: Lippincott Williams and Wilkins, 2001).

25. American College of Obstetricians and Gynecologists, *Exercise During Pregnancy and the Postpartum Period* (Technical Bulletin #189) (Washington, DC: ACOG, 1994).

26. D. E. Corbin, "Exercise Programming for Older Adults," *ACSM Resource Manual,* edited by J. L. Roitman (Philadelphia: Lippincott Williams and Wilkins, 2001).

27. D. C. Nieman, *Exercise Testing and Prescription A Health-Related Approach,* (Mountain View, CA: Mayfield, 1999).

28. "FM Pulse—Number of Overweight Children Increasing," *Fitness Management Magazine,* 17:10 (Sept. 2001), 14.

29. "Make Your Steps Count—By Counting Them a Stride at a Time," *Environmental Nutrition,* 24:9 (Sept. 2001), 3.

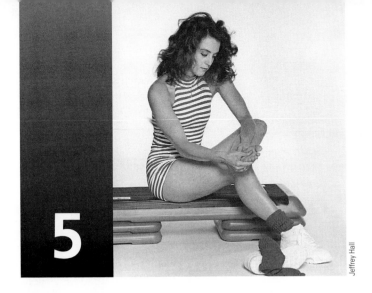

Jeffrey Hall

5

Prevention and Treatment of Walking and Jogging Injuries

Outline

Exercise participants will incur an injury or two if they exercise long enough. Fortunately, most injuries are minor and respond to minimal treatment. The aim of this chapter is to reinforce the importance of preventing injuries and to acquaint you with recognizable symptoms and effective treatments for some common injuries. The first step in treating the injury is to recognize the symptoms, and treatment should begin as soon as possible after its occurrence. In addition, certain nutritional remedies may promote the healing process and might help to prevent some injuries as well.

Principles of Injury Prevention

The often-heard adage, "An ounce of prevention is worth a pound of cure," is applicable when embarking upon a walking or jogging program. It continues to be sound advice even for seasoned participants, because after an injury-free period, some people become complacent and disregard the principles that contributed to their lack of injury. The best way to deal with injuries is to prevent them in the first place. Previous chapters have focused upon the principles of training

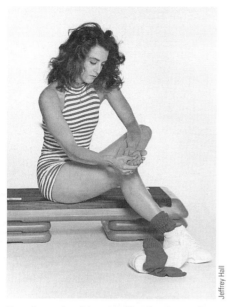

Exercisers should recognize the signs of an injury and treat it immediately.

designed to promote aerobic fitness with maximum safety. In summary:

1. Contain your enthusiasm. Enthusiasm is necessary for success, but too much can lead to overexertion and injury. You should increase the distance or decrease the time required to cover a given distance slowly and progressively.

2. If you have risk factors or are older than 45 years of age, obtain clearance for jogging by a physician.

3. Individualize your program to meet your aims and objectives.

4. Do not exceed 85 percent of maximal heart rate for the exercise intensity of each workout.

5. In the early stages of the program, keep the duration of each workout within the 20- to 30-minute range, and lengthen it as your fitness improves.

6. In the beginning, walk or jog every other day, and increase the frequency to a level consistent with physical improvement and the program objectives.

7. Wear quality walking or jogging shoes.

8. Adjust the intensity and duration of the workout according to the environmental conditions.

9. Hydrate fully prior to the workout, and continue to drink liquids during and after the workout.

10. Follow sound warm-up and cool-down procedures.

11. Work to improve your walking and jogging form.

12. Choose surfaces that are less likely to promote injuries.

Incidence and Risk of Exercise-Related Injuries

The most common exercise-induced injuries are musculoskeletal in nature.[1] Walking is a low-impact activity with an attendant low risk for injury. Jogging and running, which are high-impact activities, are associated with a higher risk for musculoskeletal injuries. Approximately 35 percent to 60 percent of runners report sustaining injuries that temporarily interrupt training, and a small percentage of these require medical treatment.[2] The most common types of running injuries are to the knees and feet and are a consequence of one or more of the following:

1. Jogging more than three times per week

2. Wearing improper footwear

3. Jogging on hard, nonresilient surfaces

4. Lack of proper warm-up

5. Overloading the muscles by attempting to do too much too soon

6. Utilizing poor form or technique

7. Jogging excessive distances

8. Jogging on hilly terrain

9. Jogging when fatigued.

Treating Common Injuries

The following discussion covers treatments for common musculoskeletal injuries associated with walking and jogging. It begins with the standard RICES treatment.

General Treatment: The RICES Principle

The standard treatment for exercise-related musculoskeletal injuries follows the **RICES principle**:[3]

R = rest
I = ice
C = compression
E = elevation
S = stabilization

The RICES techniques are designed to control the extent of tissue damage and **edema** (fluid accumulation).

Rest

The severity of an injury dictates the amount and type of rest required. Complete rest may take the form of immobilization. Active rest may rely on the use of assistive devices such as crutches, canes, and walkers. In any event, the purpose of rest is to allow time for healing without causing additional tissue damage.

Ice

Cryotherapy (the application of cold treatment) is the initial line of defense for acute injuries. The purposes of cold therapy are to decrease pain and to promote constriction of blood vessels at the site of injury, thereby controlling hemorrhage, edema, and swelling. Cold applications are thought to reduce pain either by slowing the speed of neural impulses or by overwhelming the pain receptors with so many cold impulses that the pain impulses are lost.[4]

Compression

Compression (pressure) has a twofold purpose:

1. It controls the accumulation of fluid around the site of the injury by reducing the amount of space available for swelling.

2. The compression wrap decreases extraneous and unwanted movement by the injured body part.

The compression wrap should be left in place for about 72 hours. It should not be worn during sleep and should be loosened if the injured area begins to throb or change color.

Elevation

Elevating the injured part limits swelling by decreasing the pooling of blood that otherwise would occur from the force of gravity. The veins drain blood and other fluids away from the injured area, and elevating the body part facilitates the process. The injured part should be kept elevated for most of the first 72 hours after the injury, including the sleeping hours.

Stabilization

Immediate stabilization of the injured body part through bracing and splinting supports the injured area and allows the surrounding muscles to relax. This decreases the likelihood of incurring spasms in adjacent muscles and reduces pain.

Treating Selected Injuries

The following injuries are the most common to walkers and joggers.

Achilles Tendon Injuries

The achilles tendon connects the calf muscle to the heel of the foot. Achilles tendonitis is a painful inflammation often accompanied by swelling. The three most frequent causes of achilles tendonitis are jogging uphill, wearing walking or jogging shoes with inflexible soles, and failing to maintain a stretching program. Symptoms include burning pain, which usually appears early in the workout and then subsides until the exercise ends, at which time the pain reappears and progressively worsens.

Treatment includes icing the tendon, followed by gently stretching. Prevention involves daily stretching to increase flexibility of the calf and the use of quality walking or jogging shoes.[5] Preventive maintenance is important because the tendon can tear or rupture under stress. In the latter case, surgery becomes the only effective treatment, but either situation leads to a long period of inactivity.[6]

Blisters

Blisters are painful friction burns of a minor nature that result in fluid-filled sacs of various sizes. Blisters can be prevented by wearing properly fitted shoes and clean socks and using the correct footstrike. In addition, foot or talcum powder may be sprinkled inside socks and shoes to reduce friction.

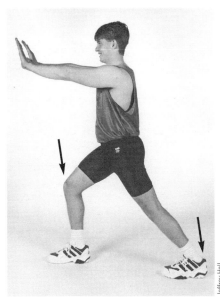

Stretching exercise aids in preventing and relieving achilles tendonitis.

Jeffrey Hall

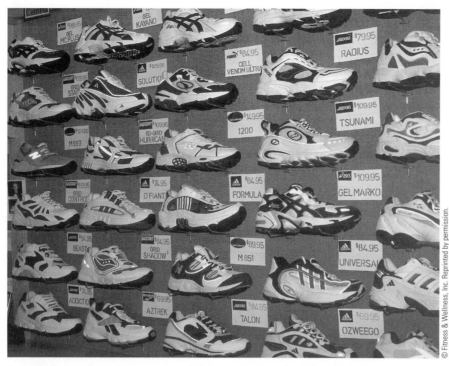

Properly fitting shoes are recommended to prevent exercise-related injuries.

Moleskin (toughskin) can be applied to areas of the feet that tend to blister. These "hot spots" are reddened areas that will become blisters quickly if preventive measures are not taken. If a blister forms:

1. Wash the area thoroughly with soap and water.

2. Apply a generous coat of iodine to the blister and the surrounding area.

3. With a sterile needle, puncture the blister at its base, and squeeze out the accumulated fluid.

4. Apply an antiseptic medication and a sterile dressing.

5. Continue exercise after treatment by cutting a "doughnut" from foam rubber and taping it over the blister.

Chafing

Chafing occurs in areas that are subject to a lot of friction. For example, people with large thighs that rub together often experience chafing. This minor but aggravating injury can be prevented easily by applying a generous coat of vaseline to susceptible areas prior to the workout. Treatment for chafing is to immediately cease walking and jogging with the onset of irritation, and to apply an antiseptic lotion.

Chondromalacia Patella

Chondromalacia patella (*chondro* = cartilage; *malacia* = softening; *patella* = kneecap) is commonly referred to as "runner's knee." This describes a condition in which the kneecap tracks laterally rather than vertically during flexion and extension of the leg. Typical symptoms are soreness around and under the kneecap, particularly when jogging uphill or climbing stairs. The pain must be eliminated before resuming jogging safely.

Treatment includes resting, applying ice, and taking aspirin every 4 hours for several weeks. Ice treatment should be discontinued after 24 to 36 hours and replaced with moist heat application several times per day as long as needed.

When pain abates, the jogger can begin progressive resistance exercises to strengthen the quadriceps group (the large muscles in the front of the thigh) and a low-intensity, graduated jogging program. Preventive measures include:

1. Using orthotic devices (supports placed in jogging shoes to compensate for biomechanical problems); these are designed to prevent abnormal motions in the foot and lower leg during jogging

2. Avoiding hard running surfaces such as concrete sidewalks

3. Abstaining from sloped or hilly terrain

4. Keeping stair-climbing to a minimum.

Hamstring Injuries

The hamstrings are a group of muscles in the back of the thigh. The muscles in this group are subject to strains and tears. There is usually a specific area of pain directly over the area of injury. Muscle strains typically occur within the belly or central part of the muscle. Severe strains occur in the tendon where the muscle originates or connects to the bones. Hamstring tears occur either high in the thigh next to the buttocks or low, just above the knee. When tears are on the inside of the thigh, they usually are close to the groin.

The RICES principle of treatment applies to hamstring injuries. The exerciser can perform mild static stretching of the hamstrings as long as this is not accompanied by pain. Forced stretches can aggravate the injury.

Iliotibial Band (ITB) Syndrome

Iliotibial band syndrome is one of the common overuse injuries among runners. The iliotibial band is a ligament that runs on the outside of the thigh from the hip to a point below the knee.[7] The band narrows below the knee and may rub against the bone, causing swelling, pain, and inflammation on the outside of the knee.

Iliotibial band injuries can occur from any repetitive activity that causes the legs to turn inward. Among the many factors that contribute to ITB syndrome are:[8]

1. Worn-down jogging shoes
2. Consistent downhill running
3. Running on banked surfaces such as a banked road that crests in the middle
4. Running too many laps in the same direction on a track
5. Jogging too many miles.

As another precaution, avoid squats. Also, a proper warm-up is important—walking one-quarter to one-half mile at a slowly increasing pace before jogging. Last, a podiatrist should be consulted regarding the possible need for **orthotics** (devices placed in shoes designed to improve the biomechanics of walking and jogging).

ITB injuries affect novice and experienced runners alike. They also are more common in women than men. This probably is attributable to the difference in hip width between men and women, which produces an angle between thighs and knees that predisposes women to injury. An ITB injury should be suspected if there is pain on the outside of the knee when it is bent at a 45-degree angle.

Treatment of ITB syndrome requires the immediate cessation of activity after the onset of pain. This may involve complete rest for a few days to a few weeks, or it may simply involve cutting back on mileage. If complete rest is the treatment of choice, non-weight-bearing exercises such as swimming, deep-water running, stationary cycling, or rowing may be substituted. If the pain does not subside after several weeks, medical attention should be sought.

Low-Back Pain

Strains that cause muscle spasms constitute 90 percent of all low-back pain. Strains are attributed to many and varied causes. Those that commonly precipitate problems for walkers and joggers are:

1. Weak abdominal muscles
2. Tight low-back and hamstring muscles
3. Overuse—increasing the mileage too rapidly
4. Faulty mechanics, particularly too much forward lean.

Preventive measures include daily stretching of the lower back and hamstrings, strengthening of the abdominals, slowly increasing the distance, and improving faulty walking and jogging mechanics. Walking and jogging strengthen the muscles of the lower back; stretching exercises keep them from shortening. At the same time, the abdominal muscles have to be strengthened because they provide some support to the spinal column in holding up the weight of the torso. Treatment of low-back pain includes rest, aspirin, and a firm mattress with a bedboard.

Morton's Neuroma

Morton's neuroma results in burning pain between the third and fourth toes, usually as a result of repetitive trauma such as that experienced by runners. Pain is the primary symptom, and it is the result of scar tissue (fibrosis) impinging upon the sensory digital nerve. The pain may be constant, or it might appear after walking or jogging on a hard surface. Narrow shoes, particularly high-heeled shoes, should be avoided.

Treatment includes the use of metatarsal bars or pads worn across the ball of the foot, shoes with a wide toe box, and local injection of a steroid preparation. Rest is suggested as long as the individual responds with pain to finger pressure at the site. If all of the above fail, surgery will be required. Prevention includes wearing walking, jogging, and everyday shoes that are roomy in the toe box, well-padded under the balls of the feet, and flexible. Walking and jogging on softer surfaces also helps.

Muscle Cramps

Muscle cramps are sudden, powerful, involuntary muscle contractions that produce considerable pain. Some cramps recur—the muscles repeatedly contract and relax—and others produce steady, continuous contraction. Preventive measures include a gradual warm-up that includes stretching exercises. Overfatigue should be avoided.

Causes associated with muscle cramping are difficult to establish. Fatigue, depletion of body fluids and minerals, and loss of muscle coordination all have been implicated.

Muscle cramps should not be massaged because of possible underlying blood vessel damage and internal bleeding. Vigorous massage in this case would aggravate the condition and promote additional damage. Treatment includes applying firm, consistent pressure at the site of the cramp, followed by the application of ice and then stretching the affected muscle.

Muscle Soreness

Muscle soreness after walking and jogging is probably attributable to microscopic tears in muscle fibers and damage to muscle membranes. This damage is partially responsible for the localized pain, tenderness, and swelling that exercisers experience 24 to 48 hours after the workout.

Downhill running and walking have been implicated in delayed muscle soreness. In downhill running, the leg muscles undergo **eccentric muscle contraction**; they produce force as they lengthen. Running uphill produces the opposite effect as the muscles undergo **concentric muscle contraction** to provide the lift needed to negotiate the upgrade.

To expand upon this concept, when a weight is lifted, the muscles contract concentrically to produce the force needed to raise the weight against the force of gravity. When the weight is returned to the starting position, the muscles contract eccentrically, lengthen, and produce the same amount of force to slow their descent. This portion of the movement is what results in delayed muscle soreness.

In a simple but ingenious study, the subjects exercised by consistently stepping onto a box with one leg and stepping down with the other. The step-up represented the concentric contraction, and the step-down the eccentric contraction. The subjects experienced pain, which peaked 48 hours after the exercise in the eccentrically exercised leg only.[9]

The delayed soreness experienced with eccentric exercise is probably attributable to the recruitment of only a few muscle fibers that must produce great tension to do the work. Untrained people have more delayed muscle soreness than trained people.

Delayed muscle soreness can be prevented by keeping the intensity, duration, and frequency of exercise within one's ability level, by progressing slowly, by doing daily stretching exercises, and by walking and jogging on a flat surface in the initial stages of training. As fitness improves, uphill and downhill walking and running are carefully introduced into the routine. Soreness is treated with rest, as well as stretching the affected muscles several times per day.

Plantar Fasciitis

Occasionally an exerciser experiences low-grade pain beneath the heel of one or both feet. In mild cases the person feels this pain during jogging, but more severe cases produce pain upon walking also. The pain results from microscopic tears and inflammation of the connective tissue (planter fascia) beneath the heel.

Treatment consists of cold therapy several times a day for the first few days, rest, anti-inflammatory drugs, heel pads, and possibly orthotic correction. Orthotics are supports placed in the walking and running shoes, designed to correct biomechanical problems. Prevention involves well-fitting, well-cushioned walking and jogging shoes and a stretching program that includes stretching the calf and achilles tendon.

Shin Splints

Shin splints produce pain that radiates along the inner surface of the large bone of the lower leg (see Figure 5.1). This condition is caused by running or walking on hard surfaces in improper shoes. It is most prevalent in unconditioned and novice exercisers who do too much too soon. Jogging or walking in one direction on a banked track or banked road shoulder can contribute to shin splints. Shin splints are the most common running injury.[10] Overweight and obesity can contribute to shin splints.

Pain associated with this injury manifests itself gradually. Initially it occurs after the workout, but as training continues, it tends to show up during the workout. In severe cases, pain accompanies walking and stair-climbing. Treatment includes rest, application of ice, wrapping or taping the shin, and placing heel lifts in the shoes.

The following exercises might help.

Toe Flexor

1. Sit in a chair with the bare feet approximately shoulder-width apart.
2. Place a towel on the floor in front of both feet, allowing the toes to overlap the near edge of the towel.
3. Repeatedly curl the toes to pull the towel toward you so it ends up under the arch of the feet.

The heels must be in contact with the floor at all times. You may place a weight, such as a book or a can of food, on the towel to increase the resistance.

Toe Extensor

This is the reverse of the toe flexor exercise. By reversing the action of the toes, you will push the towel away from you and return it to the original position. Keep your heels on the floor.

Sandsweeper

1. Sit on a chair with one bare foot on the lateral edge of a towel.
2. Grasp the towel with the toes, and pivot on the heel to the right to sweep the towel in that direction.
3. Return the foot to the starting position, and repeat until the towel has been moved completely to the right.
4. Replace the towel in the original position and sweep to the left.
5. Repeat with the other foot.

Shin splints are best prevented rather than treated. Preventive measures include wearing quality walking or jogging shoes, gradually adjusting to the rigors of training, avoiding hard surfaces and hilly terrain, using the proper heel–toe strike, and daily using the exercises described previously.

Stress Fractures

Stress fractures are tiny, often microscopic breaks in bones. The bones of the feet and shins are particularly affected. Symptoms include one or all of

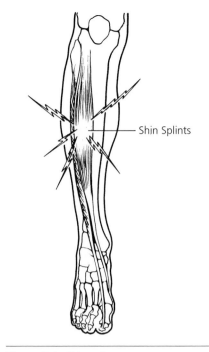

— Shin Splints

Figure 5.1 Shin splints.

the following: dull ache, local tenderness, and swelling. Pressure applied to the site of injury also produces pain.

This is a classic injury of overuse. Exercisers who are logging too many miles, exercising too often, and exercising on hard surfaces are candidates for stress fractures. Surfaces that have little or no "give" or resiliency force the body to absorb more of the shock.[11] This applies to joggers in particular because of the high shock of landing. Quality jogging shoes are a must, but they can absorb only a portion of the shock.

Women who are training heavily are susceptible to stress fractures, particularly if they become lean enough so their menstrual cycle stops, in which case the production of **estrogen** (female sex hormone) also stops. Estrogen protects the bones from thinning. A female runner who has had **amenorrhea** for a couple of years has lost a significant amount of bony tissue, and this, in combination with vigorous training, leaves her vulnerable to stress fractures. The risk of stress fractures for women can be reduced by cutting back on mileage and by not becoming so lean as to interrupt the menstrual cycle.

If a stress fracture has been diagnosed, rest is essential. The physician will advise when the person can return to physical activity. At that point, these people cannot pick up where they left off when they were injured. They should start at a low level and gradually increase the duration, frequency, and—last—the intensity of exercise.

Stretching properly before and after exercise is essential, as are walking and jogging surfaces that have some "give." Preferred surfaces are artificial surfaces (such as those found on football fields and running tracks), flat, grassy surfaces free of holes (such as public parks and golf courses), and cinder running tracks. Motorized treadmills offer a resilient surface for walking and jogging.

Other Exercise Concerns

Many joggers and would-be joggers are concerned that jogging may cause premature arthritis of the knees. After 35 years of data collection in the Framingham Heart Disease Study, the conclusion was that obesity and not jogging was the leading cause of osteoarthritis of the knees.[12] The researchers concluded that jogging was not a causative factor even in high-mileage joggers (those who jogged an average of 28 miles per week for at least 12 years). A more recent study conducted in Austria confirmed these results. An examination of marathon runners showed no long-term detrimental effects to the knees of healthy runners.[13]

A scrutiny of the research indicates that two conclusions can be drawn regarding jogging and osteoarthritis:[14]

1. The inevitability that jogging causes osteoarthritis is a myth that is not supported by the evidence.

2. Jogging can help to prevent and/or treat osteoarthritis because it strengthens the muscles, tendons, and ligaments that comprise the structure of joints.

Cartilage also responds to jogging by becoming thicker, which ultimately provides more rather than less protection to the joint.

The Wisdom of Exercising During Illness

Like everyone else, exercisers will become ill every now and then. The question is whether to exercise during these times. This depends on the severity of the illness and the extent of bodily involvement. Exercise may be continued if the symptoms are located from the chin up (runny nose, stuffiness, headache) and unaccompanied by a fever.[15] But if the illness is systemic (fever, aching joints, possible lung involvement), exercise should be suspended for the duration of the illness. Exercise can be resumed when the individual has felt well for 24 hours, but it should be resumed at a lower intensity and for a shorter duration.

Illnesses that cause diarrhea and/or vomiting, such as gastrointestinal problems and urinary tract infections, require a significant increase in fluid intake. Exercising during times when the body's fluid level is compromised should be avoided because sweating would only aggravate fluid loss and retention problems.

Mononucleosis (mono) is a viral infection that may linger for months. It is relatively common among young adult runners.[16] The most serious complication of this disease is possible rupture of the spleen. Mono has a lengthy recovery phase, so treatment emphasizes rest. This translates into no training for up to 10 weeks after the diagnosis. When exercise is finally resumed, it must be approached slowly and at a substantially lower level than before onset of the illness.

Nutritional Approaches for Preventing and Treating Illness

Many nutritionists are strongly recommending nutritional practices that may reduce the possibility of an exercise-induced injury and also may speed the recovery process.[17] These include the following.

1. Get enough calories, from a wide variety of foods, to support the energy expended during exercise, plus the energy needed to carry out other daily activities.

2. Though carbohydrate intake is extremely important and is the basis of fuel for exercise, consume at least 80 to 100 grams of high-quality protein daily.

3. Get 15 milligrams (mg) of zinc and 18 milligrams (mg) of iron each day (surveys show that walkers and joggers usually do not consume that much).

4. Take up to 1,500 mg of calcium, 400 IU (international units) of vitamin D, and 200 mg of vitamin C each day.

Once a joint is injured, it becomes more susceptible to developing osteoarthritis. In addition to the RICES procedure and other first aid that may be required, treatment may include taking glucosamine and chondroitin sulfate. Backed by research, this combination has been shown to reduce **inflammation**, improve mobility, and may promote cartilage growth. The body degrades glucosamine and chondroitin rapidly, so it is recommended that 1,200 to 1,500 mg be taken three times a day during the course of treatment for injury.

Terms

Amenorrhea	Edema
Concentric muscle contraction	Estrogen
	Inflammation
Cryotherapy	Orthotics
Eccentric muscle contraction	RICES principle

Summary

❖ Common-sense safety principles will help to prevent exercise-related injuries.

❖ The RICES principle is the general treatment suggested for many types of exercise-related injuries.

❖ The exerciser should hydrate fully prior to working out and continue to drink liquid during and after exercising.

❖ Walking and jogging surfaces affect the risk of injury and should be selected carefully.

❖ Prevention of achilles tendon injuries includes daily stretching of the achilles tendon and calf muscles, as well as wearing quality walking and jogging shoes. Treatment includes icing and daily stretching.

❖ Blisters may be prevented by wearing properly fitted shoes and clean socks, sprinkling talcum powder inside the shoes and socks, and using the proper foot strike. Treatment involves puncturing the blister with a sterile needle so the fluid can be removed and a strike bandage applied.

❖ Chafing can be prevented by applying a generous coat of vaseline to susceptible areas. Treatment requires stopping the physical activity and applying an antiseptic lotion.

❖ Chondromalacia patella may be prevented by using an orthotic device in the shoes if needed, and by reducing exposure to hard running surfaces, hills, and sloped terrains. Treatment includes rest, ice applications, and aspirin every 4 hours for a couple of weeks.

❖ Hamstring injuries may be prevented by daily stretching exercise. Treatment includes use of the RICES principle and stretching exercises.

❖ Prevention of iliotibial band syndrome includes discarding worn-down walking and jogging shoes, not jogging too many miles, and not jogging downhill on a consistent basis. Treatment requires immediately stopping activity after the onset of pain.

❖ Prevention of low-back pain consists of stretching the low-back muscles and the hamstring muscles and increasing the strength of the back and abdominal muscles. Treatment may include rest plus aspirin and a firm mattress.

❖ Prevention of Morton's neuroma entails wearing shoes that have a roomy toe box, are flexible, and are well-padded under the balls of the feet. Treatment includes the use of metatarsal bars under the ball of the foot, rest, and possible surgery.

❖ Prevention of muscle cramps includes stretching exercises and a gradual warm-up prior to exercise. Depletion of body fluids and minerals also may be involved. Treatment consists of applying firm pressure at the site of the cramps, followed by icing and stretching.

❖ Prevention of delayed muscle soreness requires exercising within one's capacity, progressing slowly, doing exercises, and avoiding hilly terrain in the early stages of the exercise program. Treatment involves stretching and rest.

❖ Preventing plantar fasciitis involves wearing well-fitted, well-cushioned walking and jogging shoes and stretching the calf and achilles tendon. Treatment consists of cold therapy, rest, anti-inflammatory drugs, heel pads, and possibly orthotic correction.

❖ Preventing shin splints requires the participant to wear quality walking or jogging shoes, make gradual adjustments in training, avoid hard surfaces and hilly terrain, make the proper heal–toe strike, and do stretching exercises. Treatment includes rest, ice, wrapping or taping the shin, and using heel lifts in the shoes.

❖ Prevention of stress fractures means avoiding overuse, as too much exercise is the cause of stress fractures. Treatment involves cutting back on mileage, doing stretching exercises, and walking or jogging on flat, softer surfaces.

❖ Evidence indicates that jogging does not cause premature osteoarthritis, even among high-mileage joggers.

❖ Exercise programs may go forward if one is ill from the chin up but they should be temporarily stopped for systemic illnesses.

❖ Certain nutritional practices may reduce the possibility of exercise-induced injuries and also may speed the recovery process.

Notes

1. J. E. Kovaleski, L. R. Gurchiek, and A. W. Pearsall, "Musculoskeletal Injuries: Risks, Prevention, and Care," *ACSM's Resource Manual*, edited by J. L. Roitman (Philadelphia: Lippincott Williams and Wilkins, 2001).

2. K. E. Powell, W. H. Kohl, and C. J. Casperson, "An Epidemiologic Perspective on the Causes of Running Injuries," *Physician and Sportsmedicine*, 14 (1986), 100–114.

3. W. E. Prentice, *Therapeutic Modalities in Sports Medicine* (Boston: WCB/McGraw-Hill, 1999).

4. W. E. Prentice, *Fitness and Wellness for Life* (Boston: WCB/McGraw-Hill, 1999).

5. Powell, Kohl, and Casperson, Note 2.

6. T. P. White and Editors, University of California at Berkeley *Wellness Letter, Wellness Guide to Lifelong Fitness* (Rebus, NJ: Random House, 1993).

7. M. Cimons, "Band Aid" *Runner's World*, 36:8 (Aug. 2001), 38–39.

8. Cimons, Note 7.

9. D. J. Newham et al., "Large Delayed Plasma Creatine Kinase Changes After Stepping Exercise," *Muscle Nerve*, 6 (June 1983), 380.

10. D. S. Fick et al., "Relieving Painful Shin Splints," *Physician and Sportsmedicine*, 20:12 (Dec. 1992), 105.

11. R. D. Chadbourne, "A Hard Look at Running Surfaces," *Physician and Sportsmedicine*, 18:7 (July 1990), 102.

12. D. T. Felson, "Obesity and Knee Arthritis. The Framingham Study," *Annals of Internal Medicine*, 109 (1988), 18.

13. "No Kneed to Worry," *Runner's World*, 36:8 (Aug. 2001), 27.

14. B. Ebert, "Sports Medicine—The Joint Myth," *Running Times*, 12:291 (Nov. 2001), 43.

15. K. Beck, "Get Well Soon: Running Through—or After—Illness," *Running Times*, 12:289 (Sept. 2001), 48.

16. Beck, Note 15.

17. L. Applegate, "Nutrition—Food Rx," *Runner's World*, 36:8 (Aug. 2001), 28–30.

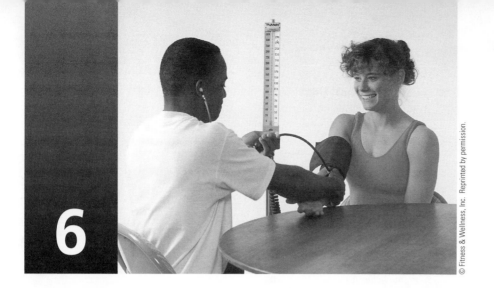

© Fitness & Wellness, Inc. Reprinted by permission.

6

Physiological Adaptations of Walking and Jogging

Outline

The human body adjusts in a number of physiological ways as it shifts gears from rest to physical exercise. Physical exertion requires prompt physiological and metabolic adaptations to meet the increase in energy demand. These adaptations are differentiated into two categories according to response and effect.

1. *Acute effects* are temporary and appear during every bout of exercise. They occur in trained and untrained exercisers alike. Normal physiology and metabolism are regained during the recovery period following the workout. The length of the recovery period varies according to the exerciser's fitness level and the intensity and duration of the workout.

2. *Chronic effects* (also known as the "training effect") are longlasting and accumulate during exercise performed consistently over weeks, months, and years. The training effects become evident during the first couple of months of exercise, and improvement in fitness continues for many years.

This chapter will concentrate on the chronic or training effects that increase physical fitness and enhance health.

Because walking and jogging often are performed outdoors, it is important to become acquainted with the environmental conditions that increase the risks associated with outdoor exercise. These will be covered in a fair amount of detail in this chapter.

VO_2 max represents the body's peak ability to assimilate, deliver, and extract oxygen and is considered to be the best indicator of physical fitness. It is a well-defined exercise endpoint that can be measured and reproduced accurately in the laboratory. VO_2 max represents the body's responses to consistent participation in **aerobic** fitness activities.

Body Size and O_2 Utilization

VO_2 max is measured in liters of oxygen utilized per minute. This absolute value is influenced considerably by body size. Because all body tissues need and use oxygen, larger people take in and use more oxygen both at rest and during exercise. Aerobic capacity, when expressed in liters of oxygen per minute, is not conducive to comparison between people, as it will yield false results. To eliminate the influence of size, aerobic capacity must be considered in terms of oxygen utilization per unit of body mass. This is accomplished by converting liters of oxygen to milliliters and then dividing by body weight in kilograms.

For example, a 220-pound person uses 4.5 liters of O_2 per minute during maximum exertion, and a 143-pound person's capacity is 3.5 liters of O_2 per minute. From these data, the larger person seems to be more aerobically fit because of a greater capacity to use oxygen. Observe what occurs, though, when these values are corrected for body size. Divide body weight in pounds by 2.2 to convert to kilograms:

$$\frac{220 \text{ lbs}}{2.2 \text{ kg}} = 100 \text{ kg}$$

Now convert liters of O_2 per minute (LO_2/min.) to milliliters of O_2 per minute by multiplying LO_2/min. by 1000 (4.5 LO_2/min. $\times$ 1000 = 4500 ml O_2/min.). Or you can just move the decimal point three places to the right to accomplish the same result.

Person A

4.5 LO_2/min. = 4500 ml O_2/min.
4500 ml. O_2/min. ÷ 100 kg (220 lbs)
   = 45 ml. O_2/kg/min.

Person B

3.5 LO_2/min. = 3500 ml O_2/min.
3500 ml O_2/min. ÷ 65 kg (143 lbs)
   = 54 ml O_2/kg/min.

From this example, the lighter person clearly can transport, extract, and use more oxygen per unit of body mass than the larger person and is better equipped to perform endurance activities. VO_2 max values expressed in ml O_2/kg/min. range from the mid-20s in sedentary older people to 94, which is the highest documented value recorded so far. This enormous capacity belongs to an extremely well-conditioned male cross-country skier. The highest value recorded for female athletes is 74, also by a cross-country skier. College-age females typically have values in the upper 30s to low 40s.

Chronic Adaptions— Training Effects

Chronic adaptations, also referred to as long-term effects, are the physiological and psychological changes that result from training. These changes represent the training effect that is developed gradually after repeated bouts of exercise.

Heart Rate

A few months of fast walking or jogging will produce a decrease in the resting heart rate (RHR) by 10 to 25 beats per minute. The decrease in resting heart rate is accompanied by a decline in exercise heart rate for a given workload. For example, a jogging speed that elicits a heart rate of 150 beats per minute prior to training might evoke a heart rate of 125 beats per minute after a few months of training. After a period of 5 to 6 months, the submaximal exercise heart rate will decrease by 20 to 40 beats per minute. Also, the exercise heart rate returns to the resting level more rapidly as physical fitness improves.

The importance of lowered resting and exercise heart rates is that this allows more time for filling the ventricles of the heart with blood to be pumped to all of the body's tissues and more time for delivering oxygen and nutrients to the heart muscle. The delivery of these substances occurs during diastole (resting phase of the heart cycle) because relaxation of the heart muscle allows the coronary vessels to open up and receive the blood they need. Training substantially prolongs the heart's **diastolic phase** with the net result that the heart operates more efficiently and with longer periods of rest.

Stroke Volume

Stroke volume (SV) and heart rate are inversely related at rest; as stroke volume increases, heart rate decreases. The heart rate at rest and the rate for a given workload are lower because of the heart's enhanced ability to pump more blood per beat. The resting and exercising heart rates are lower because training increases the stroke volume which results in the heart's enhanced ability to pump more blood per beat. This is accomplished because of more complete filling of the left ventricle combined with an increase in the contractile strength of its muscular walls, resulting in a more powerful contraction and greater emptying of the blood in the chamber. This stronger, more efficient heart is capable of meeting circulatory challenges with less beats at rest and during submaximum exercise. Training significantly increases the maximum stroke volume. In fact, the single greatest difference in the performance of untrained people and endurance-

trained people is the size of the stroke volume.

Cardiac Output

Post-training **cardiac output (Q)** increases considerably during maximum exercise, but it changes little during rest or submaximal work, primarily because the trained individual is able to extract more oxygen from the blood. The oxygen concentration in arterial blood is essentially unchanged, but the extraction rate (a-vO_2 difference) might increase significantly. With training, the a-vO_2 difference increases, resulting in more oxygen being used, as reflected by less oxygen in the venous blood. The increase in cardiac output during maximum exercise represents another major difference between untrained and endurance-trained people.[1]

Blood Pressure

High **blood pressure** is a major risk factor for heart disease. To lower the risk, elevated blood pressure has to be reduced. The vast majority of high blood pressure (90 percent to 95 percent of the cases) is categorized as **essential hypertension**. *Essential* is a medical term meaning that the cause is unknown. **Hypertension** is the medical term for high blood pressure. Although essential hypertension has no cure, it can be treated and controlled successfully.[2]

Exercise is one of the important behavioral factors that has the potential to prevent and treat established hypertension. After examining years of research evidence, the American College of Sports Medicine has drawn the following conclusions regarding the relationship between exercise and high blood pressure:[3]

1. Endurance exercise training reduces blood pressure by about 10 mmHg (millimeters of mercury) in individuals who have mild hypertension (140/90 mmHg to 180/105 mmHg).

2. Lower-intensity exercise, 40 percent to 70 percent of aerobic capacity,

seems to reduce blood pressure as much or more than higher-intensity exercise.

3. Physically active and aerobically fit hypertensives have substantially lower death rates than physically inactive hypertensives. Aerobic exercise tends to nullify many of the harmful effects of hypertension.

Scientists have yet to identify all of the mechanisms through which exercise lowers blood pressure, but the following probably are involved:[4]

1. Norepinephrine is a vasoconstrictor that clamps down on the blood vessels, increases resistance to blood flow, and raises blood pressure. Exercise lowers the level of this hormone in the blood, reduces resistance to blood flow, and lowers blood pressure.

2. Exercise likely increases vasodilator substances that dilate or open up blood vessels, decreasing resistance to blood flow.

3. Exercise stimulates the kidneys to reduce the sodium level in the blood, which in turn lowers the blood pressure.

4. Exercise contributes to weight loss, which is one of the most effective nonpharmacological means to lower blood pressure.

Blood Volume

Blood volume increases with endurance training. The volume changes from a significant increase in the amount of plasma (liquid portion of the blood) and a lesser increase in blood solids (primarily the number of red blood cells). The increase in plasma volume versus red blood cells is disproportionate. The greater increase in plasma volume results in less viscous blood that is thinner (more watery). This is an important adaptation to training because thinner blood can be circulated more efficiently and with less resistance.

A trained person's red blood cell count usually is below average, so the

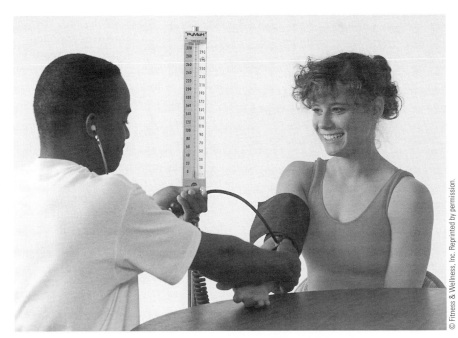

Normal apparatus and technique for measuring blood pressure.

individual could appear to be anemic. In reality, trained people have a higher absolute number of red blood cells than untrained people, but on a relative basis, because of the expanded plasma volume, the numbers seem to be low. The average **hematocrit** (ratio of red blood cells to plasma volume) of the general public is 40 percent to 50 percent. Males have slightly higher values (more red blood cells per unit of blood) than females.

The lower hematocrit of trained people is an important adaptation for endurance performance and also represents a healthy change. The ideal hematocrit for running a marathon is about 50 percent, but for health it probably is closer to 40 percent for men and 35 percent for women.[5]

Heart Volume

The heart reacts to persistent walking or jogging in much the same manner as the other muscles of the body do. It becomes stronger and, often, larger. The volume, as well as the weight of the heart, increases with endurance training. Bed rest produces the opposite effect; the heart shrinks in size.

In the not-so-distant past, exercise-induced changes in the heart were considered to be pathological. The term "athlete's heart" was assigned to describe the cardiac **hypertrophy** (heart enlargement) seen in many athletes, with the connotation that such a heart was harmful to health and longevity. Today, the medical community accepts these changes as normal responses to endurance training that have no long-term detrimental effects. In fact, maintaining such a heart for as long as possible would be beneficial. Six months of inactivity following a training program will reduce heart weight and size to pretraining levels. The **atrophy** associated with inactivity is unavoidable.

Respiratory Responses

Some training-induced adaptations also occur in the respiratory system. The muscles that support breathing improve in both strength and endurance. This increases the amount of air that can be expired after a maximum inspiration (vital capacity) and decreases the amount of air remaining in the lungs (residual volume). As a result of training, **ventilation** decreases slightly for a given workload and increases significantly during maximum exercise. This indicates an improvement in efficiency of the system. The depth of each breath (tidal volume) also increases during vigorous exercise.

Training increases blood flow in the lungs. In the sitting or standing position, many of the pulmonary capillaries in the upper regions of the lungs close down because gravity pulls blood down to the lower portions of the lungs. Exercise forces blood into the upper lobes and creates a greater surface area for the diffusion of oxygen from the alveoli (air sacs) to the pulmonary blood. This perfusion of the upper lobes of the lungs is improved with training.

Metabolic Responses

Endurance training improves aerobic capacity (VO_2 max) by 5 percent to 30 percent.[6] The magnitude of the increase depends primarily upon the initial level of fitness. Those who are the least fit make the most improvement simply because they are farthest from their genetic potential.

Fitness gains come rather quickly during the first few months of training, and further increases occur in smaller increments as fitness improves until VO_2 max reaches its peak, after 6 months to 2 years (see Figure 6.1).

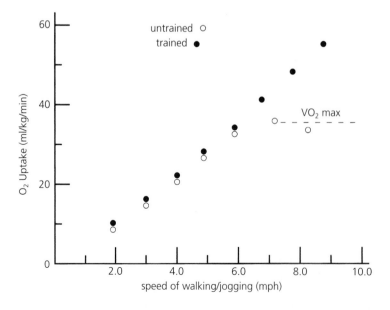

Figure 6.1 VO_2 max of trained and untrained people.

Improvement in VO_2 max results from a combination of physiological adaptations.

1. The number and size of mitochondria increase. The mitochondria (often referred to as the cells' powerhouse) are organelles within the cells that utilize oxygen to produce the ATP (adenosine triphosphate) the muscles need. ATP is a high-energy compound that provides the fuel the body uses.

2. Enzymes located within the mitochondria that accelerate the chemical reactions needed for the production of ATP are increased. These increases in the mitochondria and their enzymes produce more energy and improvement in physical fitness.

3. Maximal cardiac output and local blood supply in the exercising muscles increase.

4. The exercising muscles extract more oxygen from the blood. At rest, the arteries carry approximately 20 ml O_2 per 100 ml of blood. The veins carry about 15 ml O_2 per 100 ml of blood. When the oxygen value in the veins is subtracted from the oxygen value in the arteries, it yields the amount of oxygen the body uses. This value is termed the arterial-venous oxygen difference (a–vO_2 diff), and at rest it is equal to 5 ml O_2/100 ml blood. Because exercise increases the body's need for oxygen, the extraction rate increases and the a-vO_2 difference widens. Training increases the a-vO_2 difference during maximum exercise but does not increase it at rest or during submaximum exercise.

O_2 Deficit/O_2 Debt

When exercise begins, a short interval of time is needed for the body to adjust to the increased oxygen demand. This period, when the oxygen demand of exercise exceeds the body's transport capability, is referred to as the **oxygen deficit**, as illustrated in Figure 6.2.

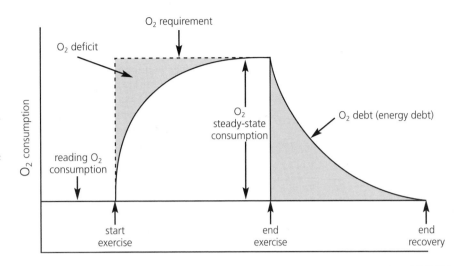

Figure 6.2 The O_2 deficit and O_2 debt.

A second phenomenon—**oxygen debt**—which has been referred to more recently as "elevated postexercise oxygen consumption" (EPOC)[7] occurs during both aerobic and anaerobic exercise (see Figure 6.2). Oxygen debt refers to the amount of oxygen consumed during the exercise recovery period above that normally consumed while at rest. It is measured at the end of exercise and includes the oxygen deficit.[8]

During **anaerobic** exercise, the body cannot supply all the oxygen needed, resulting in a deficiency between supply and demand that must be repaid at the end of exercise. A 10-second sprint or running up two or three flights of stairs elevates the heart rate and ventilation. Both persist for a few moments following the activity before gradually returning to resting levels. The extra oxygen consumed during this interval represents the oxygen debt.

Aerobic exercise also produces an oxygen debt that may be entirely attributed to the oxygen deficit, particularly in low-intensity exercise. Aerobic exercise in excess of 50 percent of the aerobic capacity will produce lactic acid and a further increase in oxygen debt. Prolonged aerobic exercise well within the capacity of the performer will cause a slight increase in oxygen consumption known as **oxygen drift.**[9] There is a slow steady upward drift in oxygen consumption that may result from a combination of increased muscle temperature and circulating levels of catecholamine hormones (epinephrine and norepinephrine).

Effects of Age on VO$_2$ max

The decline in VO$_2$ max seems to parallel the functional losses as people age. Maximum heart rate, cardiac output, stroke volume, and **metabolism** decrease during the adult years. Body composition changes as muscle tissue is lost, thereby decreasing the body's energy-producing machinery. An increase in fat tissue is an impediment to physical performance.[10]

Breathing capacity decreases as the thoracic cage (chest) loses some of its elasticity, caused by weakened intercostal muscles (muscles between the ribs), increased residual volume (air remaining in the lungs after expiration), and increased rigidity of lung structures. These changes can be delayed significantly by consistent participation in exercise and physical activity.[11]

Researchers at San Diego State University studied the effect of exercise on 15 men who walked, jogged, swam, and cycled 3 to 4 days per week for 23 years.[12] The men averaged 45 years of age at the start of the study and 68 years at the 23-year mark. Their VO$_2$ max declined 13 percent during the 23 years, equivalent to a 5 percent reduction per decade in VO$_2$ max, compared to sedentary adults, whose expected loss per decade approximates 9 percent to 15 percent.[13]

Physically fit 60-year-olds have an aerobic capacity equal to unfit people who are 35 years younger. Physical training delays the deterioration often associated with aging. Current evidence suggests that at least 50 percent of the changes attributed to aging (weight gain, stooped posture, loss of muscle mass and strength, loss of energy) actually are attributable to a decline in physical activity. These physical changes are characterized by the term **disuse atrophy**. The average

loss in VO$_2$ max as people age is a gradual but systematic 1 percent per year after 20 years of age.[14]

The researchers concluded that the 13 percent loss in VO$_2$ max for the exercise group represented a true effect of aging. If the aging effect (13 percent decline) is factored out of the decline of the nonexercisers, two-thirds of their decrease in VO$_2$ max results from inactivity rather than aging.

This important long-term study has provided evidence to support what many exercisers and researchers already knew by logical deduction and anecdotal evidence: that physical training delays the deterioration of aerobic capacity at least until people reach their 60s.

Effect of Inherited Factors

Aerobic capacity is finite. Each of us is endowed with an aerobic potential limited by our heredity. A small percentage of people inherit the potential to achieve amazing feats of endurance, as exemplified by performances in marathons, ultramarathons, Iron Man triathalons, cross-country runs lasting weeks or months, and long-distance bike races. Although most of us are in the average category for aerobic capacity, we can achieve our potential with endurance training.

Researchers have attempted to quantify the influence of heredity as a component of VO$_2$ max. How much of the variability seen among people in VO$_2$ max comes from inherited factors? Although this line of inquiry is yet to be fully resolved, the differences observed between identical twins, fraternal twins, and other siblings have provided some clues. The best available evidence suggests that the genetic component represents a range of 40 percent to 66 percent of the known factors regarding the achievable VO$_2$ max for any individual.[15]

Individuals who have inherited superior cardiorespiratory endowment have the physical structure to benefit maximally from training and could become national or world-class performers if they were to train diligently and intelligently. Those who are endowed to a lesser extent (the majority of people) also can benefit from training. Although they do not have the foundation to become high-level competitors, they can train to their potential and enjoy their own accomplishments.

Effects of Gender on VO$_2$ max

Gender differences in aerobic capacity become evident after puberty, when females exhibit lower VO$_2$ values. The difference is attributed to smaller heart size per unit of body weight, less oxygen-carrying capacity because of lower blood hemoglobin concentration, less muscle tissue, and more body fat.[16] The sexes overlap considerably regarding aerobic capacity, though. World-class females competing in endurance events are aerobically superior to most males, but they have lower values than world-class male competitors.

The differences between males and females are probably a combination of true physiological limitations and cultural restraints that have been placed upon females regarding endurance training and competition. The influence of culture and biology on female performance eventually will become clearer as more females train and compete during the next decade. Evidence indicates, however, that males and females respond to training in a similar manner and experience the same percentage of VO$_2$ improvement.[17]

Anaerobic Threshold— Lactate Threshold

Even though VO$_2$ max reaches a peak early in the training program, aerobic performance continues to improve for many years with harder and continued training. The question, then, is how physical performance can continue to improve after VO$_2$ max has leveled off. This can be answered by using an example.

Let us assume that a female jogger has achieved her aerobic potential of 54 ml/kg/min. after 2 years of regular training. At this point she is able to jog a 5-mile course at 38 ml/kg/min., or 70 percent of her aerobic capacity. After 2 more years of vigorous training (VO$_2$ max still at 54 ml/kg/min.), she now is able to sustain a 47 ml/kg/min. pace for the same distance, or 88 percent of her aerobic capacity. The past 2 years of training have permitted her to use more oxygen, thereby sustaining a faster pace for the course without dipping materially into the anaerobic fuel systems that produce lactic acid and oxygen debt.

The point during exercise at which blood lactate suddenly begins to increase is defined as the **anaerobic threshold** or **lactate threshold**. Training moves the anaerobic threshold closer to the VO$_2$ max, allowing people to exercise at a higher percentage of their capacity before lactic acid accumulates to the point at which it begins to interfere with muscle contraction and physical performance. Two people with the same VO$_2$ max will perform differently in an endurance event if one has an anaerobic threshold substantially higher than the other.

Although VO$_2$ max is recognized as an important predictor of endurance performance, several recent studies have suggested that the highest percentage of the aerobic capacity that can be sustained over an extended period of effort without a significant increase in blood lactic acid might be an even more important predictor of aerobic performance.[18]

Deconditioning— Losing the Training Effect

Deconditioning takes place when training is discontinued or significantly reduced. E. F. Coyle investigated the physiological changes that accompany detraining, as well as the approximate timetable of their occurrence.[19] The subjects in this study had been actively training for 10 years. They abandoned training for 84 days (12 weeks) so

Coyle could observe and measure the changes that took place. Coyle noted that some systems of the body showed the effects of detraining rapidly, whereas others reacted more slowly.

Stroke volume declined substantially in the first 12 days. As expected, the decline was accompanied by a significant reduction in aerobic capacity, which declined 16 percent by the 56th day of the deconditioning period. The oxidative enzyme level in the muscles had dropped 40 percent by the end of 8 weeks. By the end of the detraining period, however, the capillary density of the muscles had declined by only 7 percent below the trained state, and mitochondrial enzymes remained 50 percent higher than those of the sedentary control subjects. As a result of detraining, both heart muscle mass and blood volume also decreased.

Walking/Jogging in Various Climatic Conditions

Human beings are compelled to function in a variety of environmental conditions. People live and work in frigid, temperate, and tropical zones, at sea level and at high altitudes, and have adapted and learned to tolerate extremes in temperature. In cold weather, body temperature can be maintained by putting on more clothes or by increasing the body's production of heat through physical movement or shivering. In hot environments, heat is lost through sweating, increasing the blood flow to the skin, or by wearing as little clothing as the law and culture will allow.

Hot Weather

Humans are homeotherms (meaning "same heat"), capable of maintaining the constant internal temperature necessary to support life-sustaining processes such as cellular metabolism, oxygen transport, and muscular contraction. We exist within a relatively narrow band of internal temperature, ranging from 97 to 99 degrees F.,

although our temperature can (and often does) rise to 104 degrees during exercise.

Body temperatures that rise above 106 degrees, if not rapidly reduced, can result in cellular deterioration, permanent brain damage, and death. Temperatures below 93 degrees slow metabolism to the extent that unconsciousness and cardiac arrhythmias (disturbances of normal heart rhythm that can be fatal) are likely.

The body produces heat as a byproduct of metabolism. Physical activities increase metabolism significantly, generating more heat than normal. During physical activity only 25 percent of the metabolic energy expended actually supports the work, while the remaining 75 percent is released as heat in the contracting muscles.[20] If heat is not dissipated effectively, **hyperthermia** (abnormally high body temperature) can result in illness and possible death.

Heat exhaustion is a serious condition but not an imminent threat to life. It is characterized by dizziness, fainting, rapid pulse, and cool skin. Treatment includes immediately ceasing activity and moving to a cool, shady place. The victim is placed in a reclining position and given cool fluids to drink.

Heat stroke, the most severe of the heat-induced illnesses, is a medical emergency and a threat to life. Symptoms include high temperature (approximately 104 degrees F or above) and dry skin, caused when sweating stops. These symptoms are accompanied by some or all of the following: delirium, convulsions, and loss of consciousness. Early warning signs include chills, nausea, headache, and general weakness. Victims of heat stroke should be rushed to the nearest hospital immediately for treatment.

Mechanisms of Heat Loss and Heat Transfer

Heat is lost from the body by conduction, radiation, convection, and evaporation of sweat. Conduction, convection, and radiation are mechanisms responsible for heat transfer. The weather conditions determine through these mechanisms whether walkers and joggers lose or gain heat. Evaporation of sweat is a true heat-loss mechanism because the transfer of heat can travel in only one direction —from the body to the environment.

1. *Conduction.* **Conduction** occurs when two objects, one cooler than the other, come into direct physical contact. The greater the difference in temperature between the objects, the greater is the transfer of heat. If you enter an air-conditioned room from outdoors on a summer day and sit in a cool leather chair, you will lose heat through contact with the cooler chair.

Conductive heat loss occurs even more rapidly in water. Water is a conductor. It absorbs several thousand times more heat than does air at the same temperature. This is the reason that sitting at the poolside is more comfortable than sitting in the pool, even if the air and water temperatures are equal.

2. *Convection.* Heat loss by **convection** occurs when a gas or liquid that is cooler than the body moves across the skin. If the gas or liquid is warmer than the skin temperature, the body will accept heat rather than lose it. This occurs at about 95 degrees Fahrenheit (F). If the air temperature is lower than 95 degrees F, some heat will be lost by convection.[21]

Convective heat loss from the body to the environment increases if a cool breeze is blowing, whether it is induced naturally or is caused by an electric fan. Convective heat loss accelerates if the body is immersed in cool water. Swimming is more effective than floating for heat loss because of the flow of water over the body. When one participates in water activities, convective heat loss is augmented by conductive heat loss. Heat-loss and heat-transfer mechanisms do not function in isolation; they often work together to rid the body of heat.

3. *Radiation.* Heat is lost through **radiation** because humans, animals, and inanimate objects constantly emit heat by electromagnetic waves to cooler objects in the environment. This occurs without physical contact between objects. Heat is simply transferred on a temperature gradient from warmer objects to cooler ones.

Heat loss by radiation is highly effective when the air temperature (ambient temperature) is well below skin temperature. This is one of the major reasons that outdoor exercise in cool weather is better tolerated than the same exercise in hot weather. Temperatures in the upper 80s and 90s probably will result in heat gain by radiation.

4. *Evaporation.* The primary way by which heat is lost is **evaporation** of sweat. This process is most effective when the humidity is low. High humidity significantly impairs the evaporative process because the air is already saturated and cannot accept much more moisture. High temperature and high humidity impede heat loss. Under these conditions, adjusting the intensity and duration of exercise or moving indoors where the climate can be controlled might be beneficial.

Heat loss by evaporation occurs only when sweat on the skin surface is vaporized or converted to a gas. The conversion of liquid to gas at the skin level requires heat supplied by the body. Beads of sweat that roll off the body do not contribute to the cooling process. Only the sweat that evaporates does.

Exercise in hot and humid conditions forces the body to divert more blood than usual from the working muscles to the skin in an effort to carry the heat accumulating in the deeper recesses to the outer shell. The net result is that the exercising muscles are deprived of a full complement of blood and cannot work as long or as hard. Exercise, therefore, is more difficult in hot and humid weather.

Heat loss by evaporation is seriously impeded when participants wear nonporous garments such as rubberized and plastic exercise suits. These garments encourage sweating, but their nonporous nature does not allow sweat to evaporate. This is dangerous because it easily can result in heat build-up and **dehydration**, leading to heat-stress illnesses.

Exercisers should dress for hot-weather exercise by wearing shorts and a porous top. A mesh, baseball-type cap is optional; it is effective in blocking the absorption of radiant heat when exercising in the middle of the day, because the sun's rays are vertical. When exercising during cooler parts of the day and when the sun is not shining, a cap makes no difference.

Guidelines for Walking and Jogging in Hot Weather

Guidelines for exercising in heat and humidity have been developed for road races. These can be applied to any strenuous physical activity performed outdoors during warm weather. Outdoor conditions for exercise are safe when any combination of heat and humidity fall into the "safe" category as defined in Figure 6.3. The

figure includes instructions on how to use the chart. Caution should be used when the temperature and humidity exceed these values. People who are trained and heat-acclimated can continue to exercise at higher temperatures and humidities, but they should take precautions to prevent heat-related illness.

Notice the relationship between temperature and humidity in the figure. The higher the percent humidity, the lower the temperature must be to exercise safely. Conversely, the lower the humidity, the higher the temperature can be to exercise safety.

The keys to exercising without incident in hot weather are to acclimate to the heat and to maintain the body's normal fluid level. The major consequence of dehydration (excessive fluid loss) is a reduction in blood volume.[22] This results in sluggish circulation, which decreases the delivery of oxygen to the exercising muscles. Further, lowered blood volume results in less blood that can be sent to the skin to remove the heat generated by exercise. If too much of the blood volume is lost, sweating will stop and the body temperature will rise, leading to heat-stress illness. Heat illness is a serious problem that can be avoided by following a few guidelines designed to preserve the body's fluid level:[23]

1. Hyperhydration—pre-exercise:
   a. The exerciser should remain fully hydrated between days of exercise. This involves drinking fluids often, even when you are not thirsty. Waiting to drink until you become thirsty means you are becoming dehydrated.
   b. The exerciser should drink at least 16 ounces of water, preferably more, 15 to 20 minutes prior to a workout.

2. Fluid replacement during exercise: The primary reason for drinking during exercise is to maintain body water stores so sweating can continue:
   a. Water is the preferred fluid to drink when exercise lasts less

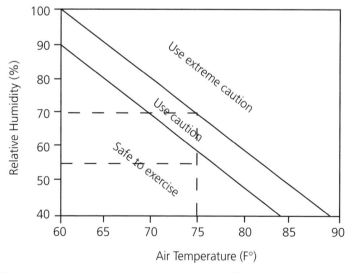

Note: There is an inverse relationship between heat and humidity. To use this chart plot the intersection between the heat and humidity. For example: If the temperature is 75 degrees and the humidity is 70 percent the intersect lands between "caution" and "extreme caution." But a temperature of 75 degrees is safe if the humidity is 55 percent.

Figure 6.3 Guidelines for exercise in heat and humidity.

than 90 minutes. Water exits the stomach rapidly and moves to the tissues that need it.

b. Urine production slows during exercise because fluid is used to produce sweat.

c. A beverage containing salt and sugar is preferred if exercise lasts longer than 90 minutes (for example, during marathons, long-distance cycling, and ultra-distance running events and triathalons).

d. The exerciser should drink 8 ounces of a cooled (59 to 72 degrees F) tasty beverage every 15 minutes during exercise. This should encourage consumption during exercise.

3. Post-exercise fluid replacement:

a. Post-exercise fluid should be cold (45 to 55 degrees F) because this will absorb some of the body's heat, which helps cool the exerciser, and cold water leaves the stomach more rapidly than tap water, thereby meeting tissue needs sooner.

b. After exercise the exerciser should drink 1 pint (16 ounces) of water for each pound of body weight that was lost during exercise. If the workout lasts longer then 90 minutes, the beverage should contain modest amounts of salt and sugar.

c. The exerciser should avoid alcoholic beverages and caffeinated beverages because these stimulate the production of urine. The body needs to retain all ingested fluids for the purpose of rehydration.

d. Exercisers can opt to drink fluids that contain salt and sugar. Commercial sports drinks are appropriate. In addition, they taste good, which encourages exercisers to drink more. This counteracts the tendency of most people to drink less fluid than they need.

e. For those who engage in prolonged walking or jogging

(greater than 90 minutes) in hot weather and those who work outdoors in the heat should understand that drinking water alone can have serious consequences because it reduces the body's stores of sodium. This condition is called **hyponatremia.**[24] It may involve disorientation, confusion, seizures, and coma. The beverage of choice to avoid hyponatremia—which literally means an abnormally low concentration of sodium in the blood—should contain the same proportion of sodium as that lost in sweat. Commercial drinks usually contain the correct amount of sodium.

4. Because more than 95 percent of the weight lost during exercise is fluid, weight loss becomes a good indicator of the amount of fluid loss. For estimating fluid loss:

a. Weigh yourself in the nude before and after exercise.

b. Towel off sweat completely after exercise and then weigh yourself. Each pound of weight loss represents about 1 pint of fluid loss. The exerciser should drink that and more after exercise.

5. Other considerations:

a. The exercise program can be modified by

(1) working out during cooler times of day

(2) choosing shady routes where water is available

(3) slowing the pace and/or shortening the duration of exercise on particularly oppressive days

(4) wearing light, loose, porous clothing to facilitate the evaporation of sweat.

b. Salt tablets are taboo. They are a stomach irritant, they attract fluid to the gut, they sometimes pass through the digestive system undissolved, and they can perforate the stomach lining.

c. For the average bout, the exerciser need not worry about

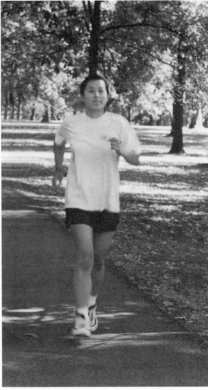

Warm-weather jogging clothes should be lightweight to promote cooling.

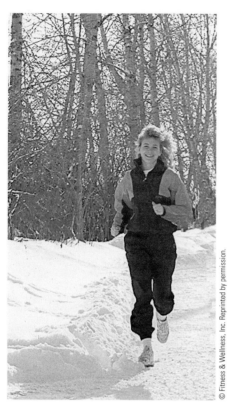

Cold-weather exercise clothing should be layered to trap and retain body heat.

depleting potassium or make a special effort to replace it. To reduce potassium stores, exercise has to be prolonged, produce profuse sweating, and occur over a number of consecutive days. Daily consumption of fresh fruits and vegetables, as suggested by food consumption guidelines, is all that is needed.

Cold Weather

Problems related to exercise in cold weather include frostbite and hypothermia (abnormally low body temperature). Frostbite can lead to permanent damage or loss of a body part from gangrene. Frostbite can be prevented by adequately protecting exposed areas such as fingers, nose, ears, facial skin, and toes. The exerciser should wear gloves, preferably mittens or thick socks, to protect the fingers, hands, and wrists. A stocking cap is recommended. Blood vessels in the scalp do not constrict effectively, so a significant amount of heat is lost if the person does not wear a head covering, and a stocking cap can be pulled down to protect the ears.

In very cold or windy weather, a surgical or ski mask and scarf will keep the face warm and will moisten and warm inhaled air. All exposed or poorly protected flesh is vulnerable to frostbite when the temperature is low and the wind chill is high. Table 6.1 can be used as a safety guide for working and exercising in cold, windy weather. Notice the relationship between the temperature and wind speed. A temperature of 40 degrees F feels like 16 degrees F if the wind is blowing at 25 mph.

People often develop a hacking cough for a minute or two after physical exertion in cold weather. This is normal and should not cause alarm. Very cold, dry air may not be fully moistened when it is inhaled rapidly and in large volumes during exercise. This causes the lining of the throat to dry out. When the person stops exercising, the respiratory rate slows and the volume of inhaled air decreases, allowing enough time for the body to fully moisturize it. Coughing stops within a couple of minutes as the linings are remoistened.

Of the problems associated with outdoor activity in cold weather,

Table 6.1　Wind Chill Index

Wind Speed (mph)	Actual Thermometer Reading (°F)											
	50	40	30	20	10	0	–10	–20	–30	–40	–50	–60
	Equivalent Temperature (°F)											
Calm	50	40	30	20	10	0	–10	–20	–30	–40	–50	–60
5	48	37	27	16	6	–5	–15	–26	–36	–47	–57	–68
10	40	28	16	4	–9	–21	–33	–46	–58	–70	–83	–95
15	36	22	9	–5	–18	–36	–45	–58	–72	–85	–99	–112
20	32	18	4	–10	–25	–39	–53	–67	–82	–96	–110	–124
25	30	16	0	–15	–29	–44	–59	–74	–88	–104	–118	–133
30	28	13	–2	–18	–33	–48	–63	–79	–94	–109	–125	–140
35	27	11	–4	–20	–35	–49	–67	–82	–98	–113	–129	–145
40*	26	10	–6	–21	–37	–53	–69	–85	–100	–116	–132	–148

Little danger (for properly clothed person)　　　　Increasing danger — cover up fully (hands, ears, face, head)　　　　Great danger — exercise indoors

* Wind speeds higher than 40 mph have little additional effect.

From *Physiology of Fitness*, by B. J. Sharkey (Champaign, IL: Human Kinetics Books, 1990).

hypothermia is the most severe. It occurs when body heat is lost faster than it can be produced, which can be life-threatening. Heat is lost primarily by convection because of the large difference between the skin and the temperature of the air.[25]

Exercise in cold weather requires insulating layers of clothing to preserve normal body heat. Without this protection, body heat is lost quickly because of the large temperature gradient between the skin and the environment. In addition to the insulating qualities of layers of clothing, a layer or two can be discarded if you get too hot.

Hypothermia can set in even if the air temperature is above freezing. For instance, the rate of heat loss for any temperature is influenced by wind velocity. Wind velocity increases the amount of cold air molecules that come in contact with the skin. The more cold molecules, the more effective is the heat loss. The speed of walking or jogging into the wind must be added to the speed of the wind chill.

The exerciser should wear enough clothing to stay warm but not so much as to induce profuse sweating. The amount of clothing appropriate for outdoor activities depends upon the experience that comes from participating in cold weather conditions. Clothing that becomes wet with sweat loses its insulating qualities and becomes a conductor of heat, moving it from the body quickly and potentially endangering the exerciser.

If you exercise or work outdoors in cold weather, you may want to wear polypropylene undergarments. Polypropylene is designed to whisk perspiration from the skin so evaporative cooling will not rob heat from the body. You should wear a warm outer garment, preferably made of wool, over this material. If it is windy, you should wear a breathable windbreaker as the outer layer. If you follow the guidelines for activity in hot and cold weather, you usually can participate quite comfortably all year long.

Assessing Cardiorespiratory Endurance

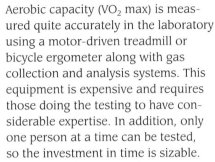

Aerobic capacity (VO_2 max) is measured quite accurately in the laboratory using a motor-driven treadmill or bicycle ergometer along with gas collection and analysis systems. This equipment is expensive and requires those doing the testing to have considerable expertise. In addition, only one person at a time can be tested, so the investment in time is sizable.

Because these procedures are inappropriate for large groups, investigators have attempted to find economical substitutes that would yield accurate results. Three field tests have been selected in lieu of laboratory tests. They correlate quite well with the laboratory tests and are easier to administer.

Walking Tests

The most used walking tests are the Rockport and the 3-mile walking tests.

Rockport Fitness Walking Test

The Rockport test estimates aerobic capacity based on the variables of age, gender, time required to walk 1 mile, and heart rate achieved at the end of the test. The course should be flat and premeasured, preferably a 440-yard track. A stopwatch or a watch with a secondhand is required. Steps in taking the test are as follows:

1. Warm up for 5 to 10 minutes before taking the test. Preparation for the test should consist of a ¼-mile walk followed by stretching exercises.

2. During the test, walk at a brisk pace and cover 1 mile as rapidly as possible.

3. Take your pulse rate immediately after the test. Count the heart rate for 15 seconds and multiply by 4 to get beats per minute.

4. On Figure 6.4 or 6.5, record the rate that is appropriate for your age and gender. Draw a vertical line

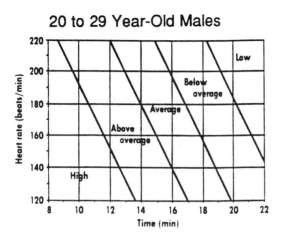

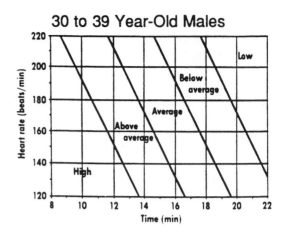

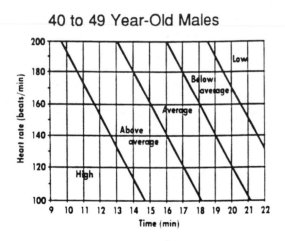

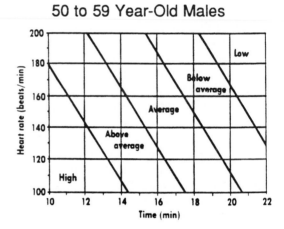

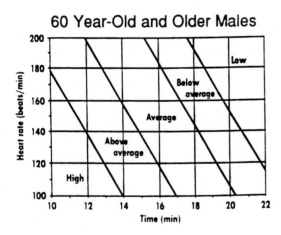

Figure 6.4 Charts for Rockport Walking test (males).

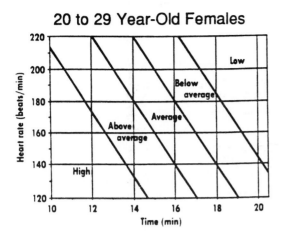

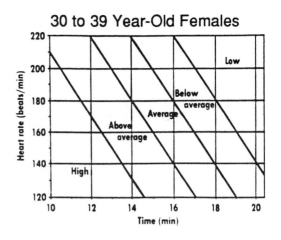

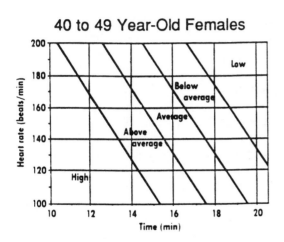

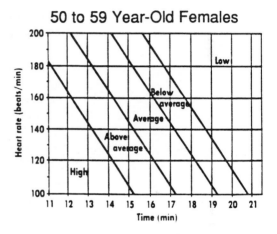

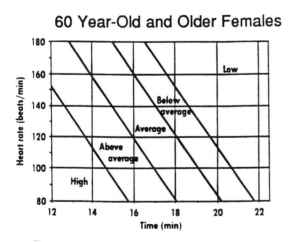

Figure 6.5 Charts for Rockport Walking test (females).

through your time and a horizontal line through your heart rate. The point where the lines intersect determines your fitness level.

These charts are designed to tell you how fit you are compared with other individuals of your age and gender. For example, if your coordinates place you in the "above average" section of the chart, you are in better shape than the average person in your category.

The charts are based on weights of 170 pounds for men and 125 pounds for women. If you weigh substantially more, your relative cardiovascular fitness level will be slightly overestimated. If you weigh substantially less, your relative cardiovascular level will be slightly underestimated.

3-Mile Walking Test

The 3-mile walking test is a test to fatigue. No running is allowed. The duration of this test and the fact that it demands a maximum effort (walking the distance as quickly as possible) requires you to train at least 6 weeks before attempting it. Students attain their best scores when they first are allowed two practice trials walking the distance. This experience enables them to find the pace that will result in the fastest time within their fitness capacity. Some suggestions for taking the test are the following:

1. Walk at an even pace, but attempt the fastest pace you can maintain for the entire distance.

2. Avoid starting out too fast. If you do, you will run out of energy too soon.

3. Rest the day before and the day after the test.

4. Eat a predominantly carbohydrate meal (pasta, rice, potatoes, pancakes) that is low in fat. Select foods that have given you no digestive problems in the past. Eat approximately 2 to 3 hours before the test.

5. Drink plenty of liquids the day of the test. Water, Gatorade™, and fruit juices diluted with half water are appropriate.

6. Warm up before the test. About 5 to 6 minutes of walking followed by stretching exercises will suffice.

7. Cool down after the test by walking at a slower pace for 5 to 6 minutes, and do the same stretching exercises as you performed in the warm-up period.

The test is best administered on a running track 1/4 mile long; 12 full laps around will complete the test. After finishing the test, record your time and compare it with the numbers listed in Table 6.2 to determine your fitness level. For example, if a 19-year old female walks the 3 miles in 41 minutes and 28 seconds (41:28), her fitness level is "Fair."

Jogging/Running Test

The best test for jogging/running is the 1.5-mile run test.

Table 6.2 Level of Aerobic Fitness—3-Mile Walking Test

Fitness Category	13–19 Yr		20–29 Yr		30–39 Yr	
	Male	Female	Male	Female	Male	Female
Excellent	<33:00	<35:00	<34:00	<36:00	<35:00	<37:50
Good	33–37:30	35–39:30	34–38:30	36–40:30	35–40:00	37:30–42:00
Fair	37:31–41:00	39:31–43:00	38:31–42:00	40:31–44:00	40:01–44:30	42:01–46:30
Poor	41:01–45:00	43:01–47:00	42:01–46:00	44:01–48:00	44:31–49:00	46:31–51:00
Very Poor	>45:00	>47:00	>46:00	>48:00	>49:00	>51:00

< = Less than; > = greater than

1.5-Mile Run Test

The 1.5-mile run has been correlated highly with treadmill tests in the measurement of aerobic capacity.[26] It has the following advantages over laboratory testing:

1. A number of people can be tested at the same time.

2. The test is easy to administer.

3. The only equipment needed is a measured course and a stopwatch.

The validity and accuracy of the 1.5-mile test can be increased by allowing those tested an opportunity to have several practice trials over the test course, spaced over a week or 10 days. Thus, each subject becomes familiar with the course and with the pace required to produce an optimal score. After several practice trials, each subject attempts to run the course in the fastest possible time within his or her capacity. The most valid results are attained when the person makes an all-out effort.

The time required to cover the distance represents the score earned. Walking is allowed if the person needs to rest but, of course, it will detract from the score, as it adds time to cover the distance. Table 6.3 translates the time taken to cover the distance into one's estimated aerobic capacity (VO_2 max). After obtaining this value, Table 6.4 is consulted for placement into a fitness category.

For example, a 22-year-old female covers the 1.5-mile distance in 13:20 minutes. Table 6.3 indicates that she has an estimated VO_2 max of 37 ml/kg/min. Table 6.4 indicates that 37 ml/kg/min. falls in the "Fair" category, but note that the average VO_2 max of females is 15 percent to 20 percent lower than that of males. Therefore, to assess this female's fitness level correctly, you must shift one category to the left, so she moves from "fair" to "average." No adjustment is needed in Table 6.4 to assess the fitness level of males correctly.

Table 6.3 Estimate of Aerobic Capacity

Time (in minutes and seconds)	Estimated VO_2 max (in ml/kg/min)
7:30 or less	75
7:31 – 8:00	72
8:01 – 8:30	67
8:31 – 9:00	62
9:01 – 9:30	58
9:31 – 10:00	55
10:01 – 10:30	52
10:31 – 11:00	49
11:01 – 11:30	46
11:31 – 12:00	44
12:01 – 12:30	41
12:31 – 13:00	39
13:01 – 13:30	37
13:31 – 14:00	36
14:01 – 14:30	34
14:31 – 15:00	33
15:01 – 15:30	31
15:31 – 16:00	30
16:01 – 16:30	28
16:31 – 17:00	27
17:01 – 17:30	26
17:31 – 18:00	25

Adapted from "A Means of Assessing Maximal Oxygen Intake," by K. H. Cooper, *Journal of the American Medical Association*, 203 (1968), 201–204.

Table 6.4 Fitness Levels for 1.5-Mile Jog/Run Test

Age Group (yrs)	High	Good	Average	Fair	Poor
10–19	Above 66	57–66	47–56	38–46	Below 38
20–29	Above 62	53–62	43–52	33–42	Below 33
30–39	Above 58	49–58	39–48	30–38	Below 30
40–49	Above 54	45–54	36–44	26–35	Below 26
50–59	Above 50	42–50	34–41	24–33	Below 24
60–69	Above 46	39–46	31–38	22–30	Below 22
70–79	Above 42	36–42	28–35	20–27	Below 20

Note: The average maximal O_2 uptake of females is 15% to 20% lower than that of males. To find the appropriate category for females, locate the score in the above table and shift one category to the left (the "Average" category for males is the "Good" category for females).

Adapted from *Training for Sport and Activity*, by Jack H. Wilmore. Published by Allyn and Bacon, Boston, MA. Copyright © 1982 by Pearson Education. Adapted by permission of the publisher.

Terms

Aerobic	Heat stroke
Anaerobic	Hematocrit
Anaerobic threshold	Hypertension
Atrophy	Hyperthermia
Blood pressure	Hypertrophy
Cardiac output (Q)	Hyponatremia
Conduction	Hypothermia
Convection	Lactate threshold
Dehydration	Metabolism
Diastolic phase	Oxygen debt
Disuse atrophy	Oxygen deficit
Essential hypertension	Oxygen drift
Evaporation	Radiation
Heat exhaustion	Stroke volume (SV)
	Ventilation
	VO$_2$ max

Summary

❖ Aerobic capacity (VO$_2$ max) is the body's peak ability to assimilate, deliver, and extract oxygen for physical work.

❖ Males generally have higher aerobic capacities than females.

❖ VO$_2$ max decreases with age, but age per se is responsible for less than 50 percent of the decline. Inactivity is responsible for most of the loss.

❖ Training reduces the resting heart rate and increases the resting and maximum stroke volume.

❖ Lower-intensity exercise, 40 percent to 70 percent of VO$_2$ max, reduces the resting blood pressure for most people by about 10 mmHg.

❖ Training reduces viscosity of the blood by increasing the plasma volume.

❖ Heart volume increases with aerobic training.

❖ Aerobic capacity can be improved by 5 percent to 30 percent with aerobic training.

❖ Oxygen deficit occurs in the first couple of minutes of aerobic exercise

❖ Oxygen debt, currently called *elevated postexercise oxygen consumption*, occurs after the bout of exercise.

❖ A longitudinal study showed that aerobic capacity decreases much more slowly for physically fit people than for sedentary people.

❖ 50 percent of the changes that occur as people age are attributable to disuse atrophy.

❖ The point during exercise at which blood lactate suddenly begins to increase—the anaerobic threshold or lactate threshold—is an important predictor of aerobic performance.

❖ Inherited factors are responsible for approximately 40 percent to 66 percent of a person's achieved aerobic capacity.

❖ The body systems decondition at various rates when training ceases.

❖ The body loses heat by conduction, convection, radiation, and evaporation.

❖ 25 percent of the metabolic energy expended during exercise supports the work, and the remaining 75 percent is released as heat.

❖ Heat exhaustion and heat stroke are serious heat stress illnesses.

❖ The vast majority of weight loss during exercise is fluid loss.

❖ The keys to exercising safely in high heat and humidity are to acclimate to the heat and to be adequately hydrated.

❖ The most common cold-related exercise injury is frostbite; the most serious cold-weather injury is hypothermia.

❖ Aerobic capacity (VO$_2$ max) can be assessed quite accurately in the laboratory but most people do not have access to these techniques.

❖ Field tests for measuring VO$_2$ max have been devised for the general public.

❖ The Rockport 1 Mile Walking Test and the 3-Mile Walking Test require only a measured course and a stop watch, and these estimate VO$_2$ max quite well.

❖ The 1.5 Mile Run Test allows people to determine their VO$_2$ max in ml O$_2$/kg/min. and it is a very good test.

Notes

1. B. A. Franklin, and J. L. Roitman, "Cardio-respiratory Adaptations to Exercise," *ACSM's Resource Manual,* edited by J. L. Roitman (Philadelphia: Lippincott Williams and Wilkins, 2001).

2. American Heart Association, *1999 Heart and Stroke Statistical Update* (Dallas: AHA, 1999).

3. AHA, Note 2; K. J. Stewart, "Exercise and Hypertension," *ACSM's Resource Manual*, edited by J. L. Roitman (Philadelphia: Lippincott Williams and Wilkins, 2001); S. K. Powers and E. T. Howley, *Exercise Physiology Theory and Application to Fitness and Performance* (Boston: McGraw Hill Higher Education, 2001).

4. Stewart, Note 4.

5. "What's the Ideal Hematocrit?" *Physician and Sportsmedicine*, 18:8 (Aug. 1990), 35.

6. ACSM Position Stand, "The Recommended Quantity and Quality of Exercise for Developing and Maintaining Cardio-respiratory and Muscular Fitness and Flexibility in Healthy Adults," *Medicine and Science in Sports and Exercise*, 30:6 (1998), 975–991.

7. S. R. Demaree, S. K. Powers, and J. L. Lawler, "Fundamentals of Exercise Metabolism," *ACSM's Resource Manual*, edited by J. L. Roitman (Philadelphia: Lippincott Williams and Wilkins, 2001).

8. Demaree, Powers, and Lawler, Note 7.

9. R. A. Robergs and S. O. Roberts, *Exercise Physiology for Fitness, Performance, and Health* (Boston: McGraw Hill Higher Education, 2000).

10. ACSM Position Stand, "Exercise and Physical Activity for Older Adults," *Medicine and Science in Sports and Exercise*, 30:6 (1998), 992–1008.

11. D. C. Nieman, *Exercise Testing and Prescription: A Health-Related Approach* (Mountain View, CA: Mayfield, 1999).

12. F. W. Kasch et al., "The Effects of Physical Activity and Inactivity on Aerobic Power in Older Men—A Longitudinal Study," *Physician and Sportsmedicine*, 18:4 (April 1990), 73.

13. ASCM Position Stand, Note 10.

14. Powers and Howley, Note 3.

15. Powers and Howley, Note 3.

16. Robergs and Roberts, Note 9.

17. Powers and Howley, Note 3.

18. B. A. Franklin, "Normal Cardiorespiratory Responses to Acute Aerobic Exercise," *ACSM's Resource Manual,* edited by J. L. Roitman (Philadelphia: Lippincott Williams and Wilkins, 2001).

19. E. F. Coyle, "Detraining and Retention of Adaptations Induced by Endurance Training," *ACSM's Resource Manual*, edited by J. L. Roitman (Philadelphia: Lippincott Williams and Wilkins, 2001).

20. T. E. Bernard, "Environmental Considerations: Heat and Cold," *ACSM's Resource Manual*, edited by J. L. Roitman (Philadelphia: Lippincott Williams and Wilkins, 2001).

21. Bernard, Note 20.

22. T. D. Noaks, "Dehydration During Exercise: What are the Real Dangers?" *Journal of Clinical Sports Medicine*, 5 (1995), 123–128.

23. American College of Sports Medicine, *ACSM's Guidelines for Exercise Testing and Prescription* (Philadelphia: Lippincott Williams and Wilkins, 2000).

24. American College of Sports Medicine, "Position Stand: Heat and Cold Illness During Distance Running," in *Sports and Exercise Nutrition,* edited by W. D. McArdle, F. I. Katch, and V. L. Katch (Philadelphia: Lippincott Williams and Wilkins, 1999).

25. Bernard, Note 20.

26. K. H. Cooper, "A Means of Assessing Maximal Oxygen Intake," *Journal of the American Medical Association*, 203 (1968), 201–204.

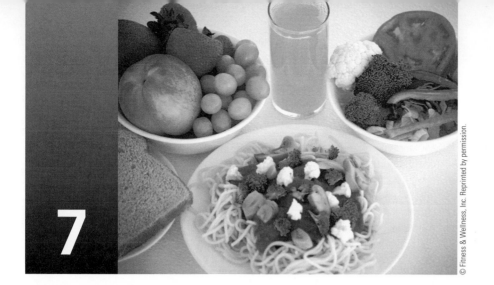

7

Nutrition for Active People

Outline

Nutrition goes hand in hand with exercise in promoting health and well-being. In this chapter we will explore how the body uses the various nutrients, particularly the energy nutrients that provide fuel for bodily activity. The discussion encompasses weight control for both overweight and underweight people, including techniques for measuring body composition.

This chapter covers the basics of a nutritious diet and the effects of diet and exercise on weight control. The **nutrients** that allow the body to perform its many functions are carbohydrates, fats, protein, vitamins, minerals, and water. They provide fuel for muscle contraction, maintain and repair body tissues, regulate chemical reactions at the cellular level, transmit neural impulses, and provide for the growth and reproduction of cells.

The roles of nutrition and exercise in weight control also are covered in this chapter, along with selected techniques for measuring overweight and overfat.

Nutrition and Health

The focus of nutrition for health changed dramatically during the last half of the 20th century. The study of nutrition during the first half of the century centered upon the deficiency diseases and their causes. After conquering these diseases in the Western industrialized world, nutritional researchers shifted their attention to the growing problem of diseases of dietary excess and imbalance.

Dietary excess is evident everywhere in the United States. Larger portion sizes of food and super-sized cola drinks are representative of unhealthy trends in the United States. Some experts are describing our current eating behaviors as indulgence in "portion distortion."[1] The impact of consuming too much food, too many calories, too much fat, not enough fiber, and not enough fruits and vegetables is reflected in the rise in overweight and obesity, an increase in the incidence of Type II diabetes, and continuing threats from heart disease, stroke, and cancer.

One of the latest investigations of trends in healthy behaviors comes from a study by the Michigan Department of Community Health and the Centers for Disease Control and Prevention.[2] The data indicated that only 3 percent of Americans were able to do all of the following: (a) maintain normal weight, (b) eat a nutritious diet, (c) exercise regularly, and (d) abstain from tobacco products. This is extremely discouraging when considering the consequences.

Obesity is a disease that coexists with risk factors for many chronic diseases and is responsible for an estimated 300,000 deaths annually.[3] A faulty diet contributes to 30 percent of all cancers.[4] Tobacco smoke contributes to more than 400,000 preventable premature deaths annually.[5] Approximately 90 percent of lung cancer, 80 percent of emphysema, 75 percent of bronchitis, and 30 percent of coronary heart disease is attributed to smoking.

Another important change in today's nutritional line of inquiry concerns the previously established minimums for essential nutrients. Many scientists are questioning their effectiveness in preventing major health problems. The Recommended Dietary Allowances (RDA) of essential nutrients has been replaced by the Daily Reference Intake (DRI), and the DRIs are being revised upward to levels that have the potential to prevent or delay the onset of chronic diseases.

For example, 60 milligrams (mg) of vitamin C was the daily requirement needed to prevent scurvy. The current DRI for this vitamin is 90 mg for men and 75 mg for women, but researchers are investigating higher daily doses (200 to 500 mg/day) and their effect on reducing the likelihood of contracting cancer and heart disease.

Another significant change in the study of nutrition involves the discovery and identification of potentially healthful chemicals found in plant foods. These include but are not limited to:

1. **Phytochemicals**, elements found only in plant foods that have the potential to prevent and treat chronic diseases

2. **Phytomedicinals**, plants that have medicinal qualities

3. **Phytoestrogens**, plant estrogens that may protect against breast cancer

4. **Antioxidants**, compounds that combat harmful elements, called free radicals or oxidants, that are the byproducts of oxidation and are implicated in the causality of heart disease, cancer, cataracts and aging.

Basic Nutrition

Metabolism is the sum total of chemical reactions by which the energy liberated from food is made available to the body. Two processes are involved:[6]

1. **Anabolism**: incorporating substances into new tissues or storing them in some form for later use

2. **Catabolism**: breaking down complex materials to simpler ones to release energy for muscular contraction.

Catabolism occurs when food is combined with oxygen. This process of **oxidation** transforms food materials into heat or mechanical energy. The energy value of food is expressed in calories. In this text we are using the term kcal, the amount of heat needed to increase the temperature of 1 kilogram of water (slightly more than 1 quart) by 1 degree Celsius. This sometimes is referred to as the "nutritionist's calorie" in that it is the unit commonly used to assign the caloric value to food.

Food Guide Pyramid

In 1992 the U.S. Department of Agriculture released the Food Guide Pyramid, shown in Figure 7.1, which replaced the basic four food groups and is a significant step forward in directing the nation's attention toward healthier eating. From a health perspective, the foods that a person should eat in the greatest quantities are the breads, cereals, pastas, fruits, and vegetables, located at the base of the pyramid. The least desirable foods (fats, oils, and sweets) are located at the apex. Each level is accompanied by the suggested number of daily servings.

Although the Food Guide Pyramid is a useful guide, it has some deficiencies, among them:

1. It gives no indication of how large a serving should be.

2. Dry beans should not be in the third level with meat because of the significant difference in fat content between the two.

3. It makes no mention of skim milk dairy products.

4. It does not differentiate saturated and unsaturated fats.

5. It makes no recommendation regarding daily fluid intake. This is an important omission because Americans may not drink enough water.

Barring these criticisms, it is a worthy guide.

Subsequent to development of the Food Guide Pyramid, the federal government stepped in and standardized serving sizes that reflect the amounts that people actually eat.[7] Before then, manufacturers were allowed to establish the serving sizes for their products. Examples of serving sizes for the various categories are included in Figure 7.1

Nutrition Facts Food Label

Since May 1994, all processed foods must display the food label mandated by the federal government. This food label is a substantial improvement over the former one in that the current label facilitates comparison of foods based on nutritional quantity and quality. The upper half of the label contains the nutritional information related specifically to the food in the package. The lower half is for reference purposes and is constant for all food products.

The upper half of the label provides the **percent daily value** for six important nutrients. The sample food label in Figure 7.2 indicates that, for example, the total fat in this specific food represents 5 percent of the daily allowance and the sodium (salt) content of this item is 13 percent of the daily allowance. The information on the upper half of the label can assist consumers in planning their daily menu without exceeding the nutritional recommendations for a given day. It also allows them to select the best foods by comparison to caloric content as well as nutrient content.

The lower half of the label provides the upper limit for selected nutrients for diets consisting of either 2,000 kcals or 2,500 kcals. The person should adjust these values in accordance with the total calorie intake.

The Calorie-Containing Nutrients

The nutrients are classified into six categories: carbohydrates, fats, proteins, vitamins, minerals, and water.

Food Guide Pyramid
A Guide to Daily Food Choices

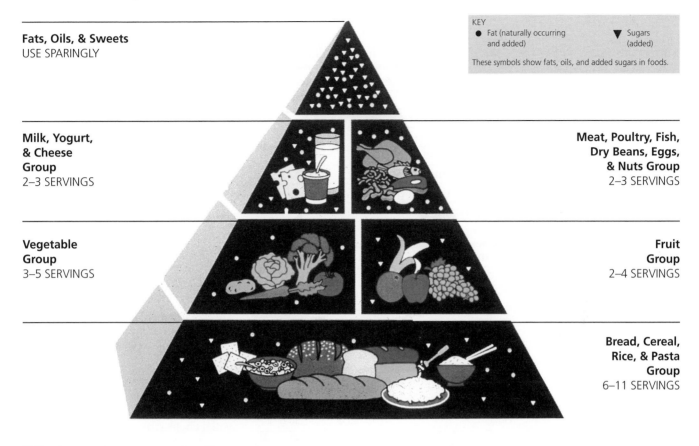

Fats, Oils, & Sweets
USE SPARINGLY

KEY
● Fat (naturally occurring and added)
▼ Sugars (added)

These symbols show fats, oils, and added sugars in foods.

Milk, Yogurt, & Cheese Group
2–3 SERVINGS

Meat, Poultry, Fish, Dry Beans, Eggs, & Nuts Group
2–3 SERVINGS

Vegetable Group
3–5 SERVINGS

Fruit Group
2–4 SERVINGS

Bread, Cereal, Rice, & Pasta Group
6–11 SERVINGS

What counts as a serving?

Grain Products Group (bread, cereal, rice, and pasta)
- 1 slice of bread
- 1 ounce of ready-to-eat cereal
- ½ cup of cooked cereal, rice, or pasta

Vegetable Group
- 1 cup of raw leafy vegetables
- ½ cup of other vegetables—cooked or chopped raw
- ¾ cup of vegetable juice

Fruit Group
- 1 medium apple, banana, orange
- ½ cup of chopped, cooked, or canned fruit
- ¾ cup of fruit juice

Milk Group (milk, yogurt, and cheese)
- 1 cup of milk or yogurt
- 1½ ounces of natural cheese
- 2 ounces of processed cheese

Meat and Beans Group (meat, poultry, fish, dry beans, eggs, and nuts)
- 2–3 ounces of cooked lean meat, poultry, or fish
- ½ cup of cooked dry beans or 1 egg counts as 1 ounce of lean meat. 2 tablespoons of peanut butter or ⅓ cup of nuts count as 1 ounce of meat.

*Some foods fit into more than one group. Dry beans, peas, and lentils can be counted as servings either in the meat and beans group or the vegetable group. These "crossover" foods can be counted as servings from either one or the other group, but not both.

Source: U.S. Dept. of Agriculture and U.S. Dept. of Health and Human Services, *Nutrition and Your Health: Dietary Guidelines for Americans* (Washington DC: U.S. Government Printing Office, 1996). (Home and Garden Bulletin No. 232).

Figure 7.1 Food Guide Pyramid.

Nutrition facts
Serving size 1/2 cup (114 g)
Servings per container 4

Amount per serving

Calories 90   Calories from fat 30

	Percent Daily Value *
Total fat 3 g	5%
Saturated fat 0 g	0%
Cholesterol 0 mg	0%
Sodium 30 mg	13%
Total carbohydrate 13 g	4%
Dietary fiber 3 g	12%
Sugars 3 g	
Protein 3 g	

Vitamin A	80%	Vitamin C	60%
Calcium	4%	Iron	4%

*Percent Daily Values are based on a 2,000 calorie diet. Your daily values may be higher or lower depending on your calorie needs:

	Calories	2,000	2,500
Total fat	Less than	65 g	80 g
Saturated fat	Less than	20 g	25 g
Cholesterol	Less than	300 mg	300 mg
Sodium	Less than	2,400 mg	2,400 mg
Total carbohydrate		300 g	375 g
Fiber		25 g	30 g

Calories per gram:
Fat   9   Carbohydrates   4   Protein   4

Figure 7.2
Sample nutrition facts food label.

The first three are referred to as the "energy nutrients," and the last three as the "regulatory nutrients."

Carbohydrates

Carbohydrates are organic compounds composed of one or more sugars (saccharides) that are derived from plants. Carbohydrates consist of monosaccharides (simple sugars), disaccharides (combination of two simple sugars), and polysaccharides (the joining of three or more simple sugars to form starch and glycogen).

Examples of simple sugars are table sugar, corn syrup, molasses, and honey. People in the United States, active and inactive alike, consume too much of these substances. Simple sugar consumption has been rising steadily. The average consumption in 1986 was 128 pounds per person; by 1996, sugar consumption had increased to 152 pounds per person.[8]

Most of the sugar intake in the United States is hidden in processed foods, the biggest offender of which is soft drinks. Americans spent $54 billion on soft drinks in 1997.[9] We currently are consuming soft drinks at a rate double that of milk and nearly six times that of fruit juices. A 12-ounce can of non-diet cola has about 10 teaspoons of sugar and 150 calories. This has prompted many nutritional authorities to refer to soft drinks as "liquid candy." Large amounts of sugar also are added to ice cream, candy, pastries, canned meats, canned soups and vegetables, and other canned products. Simple sugars are considered "empty calories," as the 112 calories per ounce they produce have little, if any, nutritional value.

Many authorities believe the excessive consumption of simple sugars leads to obesity, Type II diabetes, elevated cholesterol, heart disease, and dental caries (cavities), although the bulk of the evidence does not support most of these assumptions.[10] According to the American Dietetic Association, sugar has been erroneously indicted as the cause of a number of health problems.[11] Sugar is not an independent risk factor for any disease, except in the case of a few rare heredity disorders. For people who are insulin-resistant, however, sugar consumption increases the risk for heart disease by raising blood triglyceride levels. Also, it is a major cause of tooth decay. Sugar should constitute less than 10 percent of the total calories. Table 7.1 gives the current and recommended consumption of the carbohydrates and other energy nutrients.

The bulk of carbohydrates consumed should come from the complex form. These include starch and several forms of fiber. The complex carbohydrates are **nutrient-dense** for the number of calories they contain. This category of food is precisely what weight- and health-conscious people need. Today's dictum for health and weight control is: Lower the fat content of the diet. Increasing the intake of complex carbohydrates is a painless way to do this. Starchy foods—grains, legumes, tubers, and pastas—are both healthy and tasty. All starches come from plant foods, most of which contain only trace amounts of fat. Exceptions include olives, avocados, nuts, seeds, and coconuts, which contain substantial amounts of fat and therefore should be consumed in moderation.

Table 7.1 The Energy Nutrients—Current and Recommended Consumption

Food Category	Current Consumption (% of total Kcals)	Recommended Consumption (% of total Kcals)
Carbohydrates	50%	55–60%
	18% sugars	<10% simple sugars*
Fats	33%	25–30%**
	12% Sat fat	<8% Sat. fat*
	10% Mono	10–15% Mono
	10% Poly	10% Poly
Proteins	16%	15%

*Less than
**Fats may be as high as 35% as long as the extra 5% comes from monounsaturates and polyunsaturates.

Sources: Data compiled from: Editors, "Revised Cholesterol Guidelines," *Harvard Heart Letter*, 11:11 (2001), 6–7; Editors, "Chewing the Fats: AHA Conference Prompts New Look at Monos, Polys, Trans," *Environmental Nutrition*, 23:7 (2000), 1, 6.

Dietary Fiber

A diet high in plant foods also will be high in fiber. Processing and refining plant products diminishes the quantity of fiber significantly, if not totally. Dietary fiber is of two types: soluble, which dissolves in hot water, and insoluble, which does not dissolve. Both are beneficial to health but in different ways. Both are indigestible polysaccharides found in the stems, leaves, and seeds of plants.

Soluble fiber adds bulk to the stomach contents. This slows stomach-emptying and prolongs the sense of feeling full. This is especially good for weight-watchers. Soluble fiber also lowers blood cholesterol levels. Reducing body weight and cholesterol lowers the risk for cardiovascular disease.

Insoluble fiber adds bulk to the contents of the intestines, thereby accelerating the passage of food through the digestive tract. Among the healthy effects are that:

1. It reduces the risk of colon cancer by decreasing intestinal exposure time to cancer-causing agents in foods. It also stimulates the secretion of mucus in the colon, which coats its walls, thereby providing a barrier to **carcinogenic** (cancer-causing) substances.[12]

2. It prevents or alleviates constipation.

3. It stimulates muscle tone in the intestinal walls, which increases resistance to diverticulosis (a condition of saclike swellings in the intestinal wall).

Most plants contain some of both types of fiber. Good sources of fiber are listed in Table 7.2.

When oxidized, carbohydrates yield approximately 4 calories per gram. Because they are oxygen-rich, carbohydrates constitute the most efficient source of fuel. They are the major energy supplier in high-intensity work of short duration and in exercise of a vigorous nature for up to 60 to 90 minutes.

Foods high in carbohydrates promote the storage of glycogen (the stored form of sugar) in the liver and muscles. Increasing the storage of glycogen enhances aerobic performance of long duration such as marathon running and long-distance cycling. People who do not run such long distances should consume a diet rich in complex carbohydrates primarily because it is a healthy way to eat. Active adults should consume about 45 percent to 50 percent of their calories in the form of complex carbohydrates and no more than 10 percent in the form of simple sugars. By contrast, people who train for and compete in prolonged endurance events should consume 65 percent to 70 percent of their calories from the carbohydrate group.

Table 7.2 Selected Sources of Fiber

Sources	Dietary Fiber (grams)	Sources	Dietary Fiber (grams)
1. Cereals		4. Vegetables (½ cup)	
Kellogg's All-Bran Extra Fiber (½ cup)	15	Sweet potato (1 large)	4.2
General Mills Fiber one (½ cup)	14	Peas	4.1
Kellogg's All-Bran (½ cup)	10	Brussels sprouts	3.9
100% Bran (½ cup)	8.4	Corn	3.9
All Bran (½ cup)	8.5	Potato, baked (1 medium)	3.8
Bran Buds (⅓ cup)	7.9	Carrots (1 raw; ½ cup cooked)	2.3
Bran Chex (⅔ cup)	4.6	Collards	2.2
Corn Bran (⅔ cup)	5.4	Asparagus	2.1
Cracklin' Oat Bran (⅓ cup)	4.3	Green beans	2.1
Bran Flakes (¾ cup)	4.0	Broccoli	2.0
Oatmeal, cooked (1 cup)	2.2	Spinach	2.0
		Turnips	1.7
2. Grains (1 ounce)		Mushrooms (raw)	0.9
Brown rice, cooked (½ cup)	2.4	Summer squash	0.7
Millet, cooked (½ cup)	1.8	Lettuce (raw)	0.3
Whole wheat bread (1 slice)	1.0		
Spaghetti, cooked (½ cup)	0.8	5. Fruits	
White bread (1 slice)	0.6	Blackberries (½ cup)	4.5
White rice, cooked (½ cup)	0.1	Prunes, dried (3)	3.7
		Apples with skin (1)	2.6
3. Legumes (½ cup)		Banana (1 medium)	2.0
Kidney beans	5.8	Strawberries (¾ cup)	2.0
Pinto beans	5.3	Grapefruit (½ med)	1.7
Split peas	5.1	Peach (1 med)	1.6
White beans	5.0	Cantaloupe (¼ small)	1.4
Lima beans	4.9	Raisins (2 tablespoons)	1.3
		Orange (1 small)	1.2
		Grapes (12)	0.5

Source: Adapted from "Getting Serious About High Fiber Cereals," by A. Klausner, *Environmental Nutrition,* Sept. 1994; and Editors, "Fiber Facts," *Nutrition Action Healthletter,* Sept. 1994.

The Glycemic Index (GI)

The glycemic index (GI) is a method for ranking all carbohydrate foods by assigning each with a number that indicates the extent to which they raise blood glucose (sugar) after they are consumed.[13] Foods with a high glycemic index move rapidly from the stomach to the intestines to the bloodstream. This triggers a rapid and abnormally large spike in blood sugar as well as the secretion of larger than normal amounts of insulin as the pancreas overreacts to a sudden surge of glucose. Insulin is needed to transport glucose from the blood to the cells.

Foods with a low GI enter the bloodstream much more slowly with a less dramatic spike in blood glucose. Possible implications are that low-GI foods may prolong the feeling of fullness after a meal; the slow emptying of foods from the intestines moderates the release of insulin, producing less wear and tear on insulin-producing cells, which forestalls the development of diabetes; and, finally, the secretion of less insulin is associated with lower levels of triglycerides and higher levels of HDL cholesterol, both of which lower the risk for cardiovascular disease.

This model sounds plausible, but the ranking of foods seems to be imprecise, controversial, and, to say the least, confusing. For instance, a baked potato, long considered to be a healthy food, ranks higher on the glycemic list than table sugar, which is about as refined as carbohydrates can get. Many similar examples indicate that the GI rating system is flawed. Scientists both pro and con, however, do agree on this: Physically active people who are at a healthy weight clear sugar from the blood at an appropriate rate regardless of the types of carbohydrates they consume, and consequently do not have an increased risk for heart disease and diabetes. Perhaps the GI controversy will be cleared up in the next few years with further research.

Fats

Fats are energy-dense organic compounds that yield approximately 9 calories per gram. They have relatively low oxygen content when compared to carbohydrates and, consequently, are not as efficient as sources of fuel. More than twice the amount of oxygen is required to liberate energy from fat than from carbohydrates. Meanwhile, we store at least 50 times more energy in the form of fat than carbohydrates. A pound of fat as it is stored in the body contains 3,500 kcals.

Saturated and Unsaturated Fats

Fats are categorized as either saturated or unsaturated according to the connections between the carbons that make up the chemical chain. A fat is

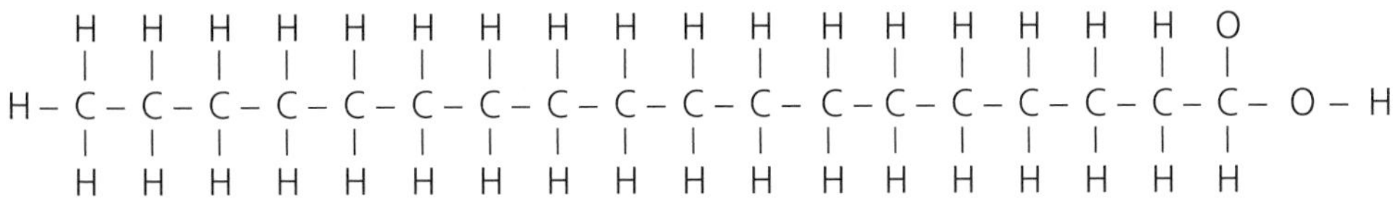

```
      H   H   H   H   H   H   H   H   H   H   H   H   H   H   H   H   H   O
      |   |   |   |   |   |   |   |   |   |   |   |   |   |   |   |   |   |
  H – C – C – C – C – C – C – C – C – C – C – C – C – C – C – C – C – C – O – H
      |   |   |   |   |   |   |   |   |   |   |   |   |   |   |   |   |
      H   H   H   H   H   H   H   H   H   H   H   H   H   H   H   H   H
```

(a) Saturated fatty acid—no double bonds: all carbons are occupied.

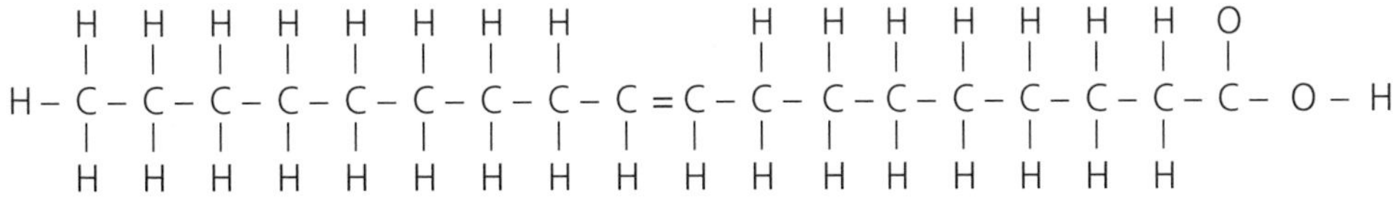

```
      H   H   H   H   H   H   H   H               H   H   H   H   H   H   H   O
      |   |   |   |   |   |   |   |               |   |   |   |   |   |   |   |
  H – C – C – C – C – C – C – C – C – C = C – C – C – C – C – C – C – C – O – H
      |   |   |   |   |   |   |   |               |   |   |   |   |   |   |
      H   H   H   H   H   H   H   H   H   H   H   H   H   H   H   H   H
```

(b) Monounsaturated fatty acid—one double bond; two hydrogens missing at that site.

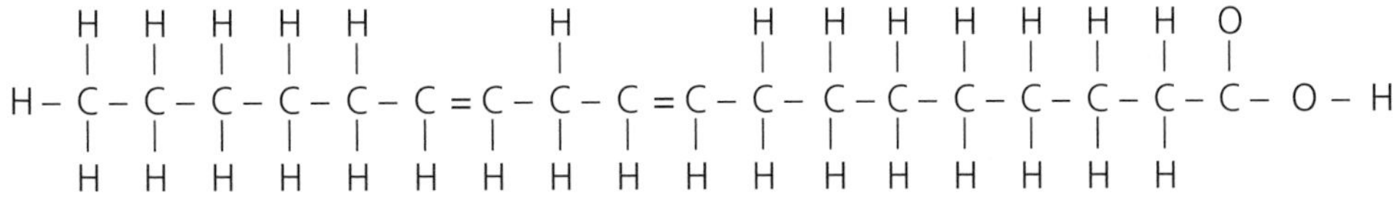

```
      H   H   H   H   H                   H               H   H   H   H   H   H   H   O
      |   |   |   |   |                   |               |   |   |   |   |   |   |   |
  H – C – C – C – C – C – C = C – C – C = C – C – C – C – C – C – C – C – O – H
      |   |   |   |   |               |               |   |   |   |   |   |   |
      H   H   H   H   H   H           H   H   H   H   H   H   H   H   H   H
```

(c) Polyunsaturated fatty acid—two double bonds; four hydrogen missing at the site.

Figure 7.3 Types of fatty acids.

saturated if the links between the carbons are single connections and all of the carbons are occupied with hydrogens. A fat is *unsaturated* if some of the hydrogens are missing, especially at sites where carbons are double-bonded. Unsaturated fats consist of monounsaturated and poly-unsaturated fats. Because all fats and oils contain a mixture of saturated and unsaturated fatty acids, the correct categorization is determined by the fatty acids present in the greatest concentration.

The most abundant of the fats, or **lipids**, are the **triglycerides**. Triglycerides make up at least 98 percent of the fat we consume as well as the fat we store. Triglycerides are composed of three fatty acids attached to a molecule of glycerol. As depicted in Figure 7.3: (a) fatty acids are saturated when all of the bonds between the carbon atoms are single bonds; (b) **monounsaturate**d fatty acids have one double bond between carbon atoms; and (c) polyunsaturated fatty acids have two or more double bonds between the carbon atoms.

The major sources of saturated fats are animal flesh, dairy products, and tropical oils (coconut and palm kernel oils). *Saturated* fats have a high melting point and solidify at room temperature. Bacon or sausage grease that stands at room temperature will solidify, signifying that it is primarily saturated. *Monounsaturated* and *poly-unsaturated* fats remain liquid at room temperature. Some food sources that are high in monounsaturated fats are avocados, canola oil, cashew nuts, olives, olive oil, peanuts, peanut oil, and peanut butter. Polyunsaturated fats are found in almonds, corn oil, cottonseed oil, filbert nuts, fish, pecans, safflower oil, sunflower oil, soybean oil, and walnuts. Some sources of plant-derived cooking oils appear in Table 7.3.

Fatty acids derived from fish, especially cold-water fish, are different from those found in vegetables and vegetable oils. The fatty acids in fish are Omega-3 fatty acids, and those found in vegetables are primarily Omega-6 fatty acids. Omega-3 fatty acids protect the heart and its blood vessels by decreasing the likelihood that the blood platelets will stick to each other. This in turn reduces plaque build-up, clot formation, and spasms

Table 7.3   Some Sources of Plant-Derived Cooking Oils

Type of Oil (grams)	Monounsaturated (grams)	Polyunsaturated (grams)	Saturated
Best Sources			
Almond	10	2	1
Canola	8	4	1
Olive	10	1	2
Good Sources			
Corn	3	8	2
Cottonseed	2	7	4
Safflower	2	10	1
Sesame	5	6	2
Soybean	3	8	2
Sunflower	3	9	1

Note: 1 gram = 1/28 ounce.

Transfatty Acids

Unsaturated fats should be refrigerated to keep them from becoming rancid. They are vulnerable to spoilage when they are left to stand at room temperature because oxygen attacks those points in the chain that are unoccupied by hydrogen. To counteract spoilage, the food industry adds hydrogen to some of the free bonds through the process of **hydrogenation**. The fat then loses its polyunsaturated characteristics, as well its health benefits.

Hydrogenation converts many double bonds to single bonds. The end product is the conversion of unsaturated fatty acids to **transfatty acids**. Margarine is one of the major sources of transfatty acids in the U.S. diet. In addition, transfatty acids are found in cookies, crackers, pies, cakes, peanut butter, fast-food fried chicken, french fries, fish—and this is just a partial list. Approximately 5 percent to 10 percent of the fat in the average U.S. diet is transfat.[15]

Vegetable oils are liquid and must be made more saturated if they are to be solidified into margarine. The harder the product (stick margarine)—versus softer margarines (tub and squeeze bottle)—the greater is the effect of hydrogenation. The question to be answered is: Does the conversion of unsaturated fatty acids to transfatty acids result in an unhealthy product? Some evidence indicates that transfatty acids have an effect similar to that of the saturated fats: They raise the blood level of harmful LDL cholesterol.[16]

Unfortunately, the food labels do not record the grams of transfatty acids found in processed foods—although this may change in the next couple of years. The Food and Drug Administration has proposed that manufacturers report transfatty acids by lumping them in with saturated fats on the food labels.[17] Second, the labels should provide separately, in a footnote at the bottom of the label, the number of grams of transfats.

Eating a fat-free diet is virtually impossible and definitely is unhealthy. The human body does require some fat. Two fatty acids, in fact, are essential. They must be obtained through the diet because they cannot be manufactured from other substances in the body. Both are polyunsaturated fatty acids that are widely distributed in plant and fish oils.

1. *Linoleic acid*, an Omega-6 fatty acid found in plants

2. *Linolenic fatty acid*, an Omega-3 fatty acid, found primarily in fish.

Proteins

Protein is an essential nutrient that yields approximately 4 calories per gram. Its energy is liberated for:

1. Building and repairing body tissues

2. Forming enzymes, hormones, antibodies, and hemoglobin

3. Transporting fats and other nutrients through the blood

4. Maintaining the acid-base balance in tissue fluids

5. Supplying energy for muscular work when there is a shortage of carbohydrates and fat.

Proteins are complex chemical structures containing carbon, oxygen,

in the arteries.[14] Fish oils are among the most unsaturated of fats, containing about twice as much as vegetable oils.

hydrogen, and nitrogen. These elements are combined into chains of different structures called **amino acids**. The proteins of all living tissue consist of 20 different amino acids. Two other rare amino acids have been identified but are found in very few proteins. Nine of the amino acids are considered *essential* because the body cannot manufacture them and they can be obtained only through the diet.

Complete proteins contain all of the essential amino acids. A high-quality protein is a complete protein that has all of the essential amino acids in amounts proportional to the body's needs for them. Meat, fish, poultry, and dairy products are high-quality proteins. Incomplete proteins do not contain the amino acids in the proportions the body needs.[18]

Plant sources of protein are usually incomplete. This is important, particularly for vegetarians, because protein synthesis is regulated by the all-or-none principle. The body cannot make partial proteins, only complete ones. Therefore, if an amino acid from a protein source is in short supply, protein synthesis will stop as soon as that amino acid is used up. Vegetarians can obtain complete proteins by consuming complementary proteins from mixing and matching foods. For example, food "A" may be missing three essential amino acids that are contained in food "B." Food "B" may be missing some essential amino acids that are found in food "A." Together, they have all of the essential amino acids. Table 7.4 offers some examples of food combinations that provide complete proteins.

Legumes, such as kidney and lima beans, black-eyed peas, garden peas, lentils, and soybeans, are excellent sources of proteins. Although their protein is not quite the caliber of meat protein, they are rich in other healthy nutrients such as B vitamins, and they are low in fat.

Daily protein requirements vary according to age. Infants require about 2.2 grams of protein per kilogram of body weight to support

Table 7.4   Vegetable Combinations That Provide Complete Proteins

Categories of Foods	Examples
Beans/wheat	Baked beans and brown bread
Beans/rice	Refried beans and rice
Dry peas/rye	Split pea soup and rye bread
Peanut butter/wheat	Peanut butter sandwich on whole wheat or whole grain bread
Cornmeal/beans	Cornbread and kidney beans
Legumes/rice	Black-eyed peas and rice
Beans/corn	Pinto beans and cornbread
Legumes/corn	Black-eyed peas and cornbread

A. C. Grandjeans, "The Vegetarian Athlete," *The Physician and Sportsmedicine* 15:191, 1987.

growth. Adolescents require 1.0 gram per kilogram. Adults need 0.8 gram per kilogram.

The typical U. S. diet contains more than adequate protein. Consuming more than 15 percent of the total calories in the form of protein seems to have no advantage. One of the major problems associated with excessive protein intake is that it usually is accomplished by increasing the consumption of animal products, which also are high in saturated fat. The increased consumption could displace fiber in the diet, and the two together can lead to a host of immediate and long-term problems.

The average daily consumption of protein by adults in the United States is about 16 percent of total calories—well above the requirement. For example, a 154-pound person requires 56 grams of protein each day. If this person is consuming 2,500 kcals/day with a typical protein intake of 15 percent, this person actually is consuming 94 grams of protein. These figures come from the following:

1. Protein requirement is calculated as follows:
   a. Convert body weight in pounds to kilograms (kg)
   $$154 \div 2.2 = 70 \text{ kg}$$
   b. 70 kg $\times$ .8 grams = 56 grams/day

2. Actual consumption is calculated as follows:
   a. 2,500 kcals/day
   $$\underline{\times .15}$$
   375 kcals of protein

b. 1 gram of protein yields 4 kcals; therefore

375 kcals ÷ 4 = 94 grams/protein

c. The difference between protein consumed and protein required is:

$$\begin{array}{r} 94 \text{ g consumed} \\ -\ 56 \text{ g required} \\ \hline 38 \text{ extra grams of protein} \end{array}$$

Many people—competitors and noncompetitors alike—who are striving to develop strength and power take amino acid supplements to build larger and more powerful muscles. Selected amino acids do not build larger muscles. Only exercise can do that. Nevertheless, these and other unfounded notions proliferate among uninformed participants who are constantly attempting to enhance their performance with substances that might give them an edge beyond what they achieve through training.

Current evidence indicates that long-distance, endurance-type athletes and weightlifters and bodybuilders have the greatest need for protein—1.5 to 1.6 grams of protein for every kilogram of body weight.[19] Even if this proves to be correct, protein supplements are not necessary, as most athletes consume more than this amount from their food intake.

Active people tend to get more vitamins in their diet than sedentary people do because active people consume more calories than their less active counterparts. If you are concerned about not getting enough vitamins in your diet but are unwilling to make appropriate dietary changes, a one-a-day brand supplemented by extra C and E should suffice.

The Regulatory Nutrients

The regulatory nutrients, which contain no calories, are vitamins, minerals, and water.

Vitamins

Vitamins are organic compounds found in small quantities in most foods. All vitamins are either fat-soluble or water-soluble. The fat-soluble vitamins (A, D, E, and K) are stored in the liver and fatty tissues until they are needed. The water-soluble vitamins (C and the B complex group) are not stored for any appreciable length of time and must be replenished daily.

Vitamins function as coenzymes that promote the many chemical reactions in the body around the clock. Because vitamin deficiencies result in a variety of diseases and adequate daily intake is necessary, the **dietary reference intake (DRI)** for most vitamins has been established. Although these amounts are needed to prevent vitamin-deficiency diseases, they do not represent optimal values.

Today, the interest in vitamins by the scientific community goes beyond that. For instance, substantial research efforts currently are attempting to clarify the role of selected antioxidant vitamins (C, E, and the carotenoids) in preventing cardiovascular disease and cancer. The early evidence is promising, and taking these vitamins in amounts larger than recommended seems to be safe.

The antioxidant vitamins protect the body from the harmful effects of **free radicals** (oxidants). Free radicals are byproducts of oxidation. Because the cells continuously use oxygen, free radicals are being produced constantly. Simultaneously, free radicals are generated by cigarette smoke, radiation from the sun and other sources, alcohol, heat, and environmental pollutants.

If free radicals are not neutralized immediately, they damage the cells and their **DNA** (the master blueprint for cellular function). Researchers estimate that each DNA of the approximately 60 trillion cells in the body takes "a hit from free radicals every 10 seconds."[20] Over the course of a lifetime, some of the cellular damage inflicted by free radicals goes unrepaired. The cumulative damage can result in the development of cancer, heart disease, cataracts, and rheuma-

Table 7.5   Toxic Symptoms of Fat-Soluble Vitamins

Vitamin (U.S. RDA)	Sources	Toxic Symptoms
Vitamin A (1000 mg)*	fortified milk and margarine, cream, cheese, butter, eggs, liver, spinach and other dark leafy greens, broccoli, apricots, peaches, cantaloupe, squash, carrots, sweet potatoes, pumpkin	red blood cell breakage, nosebleeds, abdominal cramps, nausea, diarrhea, weight loss, blurred vision, irritability, loss of appetite, bone pain, dry skin, rashes, hair loss, cessation of menstruation, growth retardation
Vitamin D (400 IU)**	self-synthesis with sunlight, fortified milk, fortified margarine, eggs, liver, fish	elevated blood calcium, constipation, weight loss, irritability, weakness, nausea, kidney stones, mental and physical retardation
Vitamin E (30 IU)	vegetable oils, green leafy vegetables, wheat germ, whole-grain products, butter, liver, egg yolk, milk fat, nuts, seeds	interference with anticlotting medication, general discomfort
Vitamin K (no U.S. RDA)	bacterial synthesis in digestive tract, liver, green leafy and cruciferous vegetables, milk	interference with anticlotting medication; may cause jaundice

*mg = micrograms
**IU = international units

toid arthritis. Free radicals also have been implicated as an agent that promotes aging.

> *People should obtain antioxidants by eating more fruits, vegetables, and whole grains.*

The antioxidant vitamins protect the cells from the damaging effects of free radicals. Many authorities, but not all, recommend taking 500 milligrams (mg) of vitamin C and 400 international units (IU) of vitamin E daily to neutralize the free radicals. All authorities agree, however, that we should obtain antioxidants by increasing our consumption of fruits, vegetables, and whole grains.

Eating these antioxidant-rich foods provides another advantage: They contain phytochemicals, which are unique to plant foods. There are literally hundreds, maybe thousands, of phytochemicals. The research that has identified these elements along with their potential health benefits is in the earliest stages of development. Thus far, the phytochemicals likely are involved in preventing cancer, heart disease, and other chronic diseases.

Continuing research will provide more answers in the next few years.

Unusually large doses (megadoses) of any vitamin are potentially hazardous. People who supplement heavily may incur vitamin toxicity, particularly from overindulgence in the fat-soluble group. When vitamins are taken in very large amounts, they cease to function as vitamins and begin to act like drugs. Also, large doses interfere with or disrupt the action of other nutrients. Tables 7.5 and 7.6 list some problems associated with vitamin megadoses.

Are synthetic vitamin supplements inferior to natural vitamin supplements? Promoters of vitamin products that come from natural sources adamantly proclaim that this is so, but in reality the synthetic and natural supplements are chemically equivalent

Active people tend to get more vitamins in their diet than sedentary people do because active people consume more calories than their less active counterparts. If you are concerned about not getting enough vitamins in your diet but are unwilling to make appropriate dietary changes, a one-a-day brand supplemented by extra C and E should suffice.

Table 7.6 Toxic Symptoms of Water-Soluble Vitamins

Vitamin (U.S. RDA)	Sources	Toxic Symptoms
Thiamin B_1 (1.5 mg)*	meat, pork, liver, fish, poultry, whole-grain and enriched breads, cereals, pasta, nuts, legumes, wheat germ, oats	rapid pulse, weakness, headaches, insomnia, irritability
Riboflavin B_2 (1.7 mg)	milk, dark green vegetables, yogurt, cottage cheese, liver, meat, whole-grain or enriched breads and cereals	none reported, but an excess of any of the B vitamins could cause a deficiency of the others
Niacin B_3 (20 mg)	meat, eggs, poultry, fish, milk, whole-grain and enriched breads and cereals, nuts, legumes, peanuts, nutritional yeast, all protein foods	flushing, nausea, headaches, cramps, ulcer irritation, heartburn, abnormal liver function, low blood pressure
Vitamin B_6 (2.0 mg)	meat, poultry, fish, shellfish, legumes, whole-grain products, green leafy vegetables, bananas	depression, fatigue, irritability, headaches, numbness, damage to nerves, difficulty walking
Folcain (Folic acid) (400 micrograms)	green leafy vegetables, organ meats, legumes, seeds	diarrhea, insomnia, irritability; could mask a vitamin B_{12} deficiency
Vitamin B_{12} (cobalamin) (3 g)**	animal products: meats, fish, poultry, shellfish, milk, cheese, eggs, nutritional yeast	none reported
Pantothenic acid (10 mg)	widespread in foods	occasional diarrhea
Biotin (300 g)	widespread in foods	none reported
Vitamin C (Ascorbic acid) (60 mg)	citrus fruits, cruciferous vegetables, tomatoes, potatoes, dark green vegetables, peppers, lettuce, cantaloupe, strawberries, mangos, papayas	nausea, abdominal cramps, diarrhea, breakdown of red blood cells in persons with certain genetic disorders; deficiency symptoms might appear at first upon withdrawal of high doses

*mg = micrograms
**g = grams

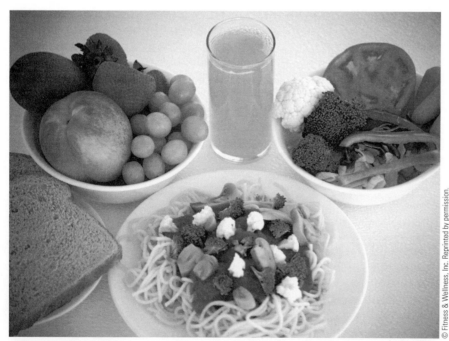

People should obtain antioxidants by eating more fruits, vegetables, and whole grains.

© Fitness & Wellness, Inc. Reprinted by permission.

and the body cannot tell them apart. Vitamin E is an exception. Natural vitamin E in supplement form is absorbed more easily than its synthetic counterpart. If a person takes 400 IU of vitamin E, it really doesn't matter whether the vitamin is natural or synthetic because the body will absorb and use more than enough.

Minerals

Minerals are inorganic substances that exist freely in nature. They are found in the soil and water, and they pervade some of the Earth's vegetation. Minerals maintain or regulate physiological processes such as muscle contraction, normal heart rhythm, body water supplies, acid–base balance of the blood, and nerve impulse conduction.

Table 7.7   Toxic Symptoms of Major Minerals

Minerals (U.S. RDA)	Selected Sources	Toxic Symptoms
Calcium (1000 mg)	milk and milk products	excess calcium is excreted except in hormonal imbalance states
Phosphorus (1000 mg)	fish (with bones), tofu, greens, legumes, all animal tissues	excess phosphorus can cause relative deficiency of calcium
Magnesium (400 mg)	nuts, legumes, whole grains, dark green vegetables, seafoods, chocolate, cocoa	not known
Sodium (no U.S. RDA)	salt, soy sauce, moderate quantities in whole (unprocessed) foods, large amounts in processed foods	hypertension
Chloride (no U.S. RDA)	salt, soy sauce, moderate quantities in whole (unprocessed) foods, large amounts in processed foods	normally harmless (chlorine gas is a poison but evaporates from water), disturbed acid-base balance, vomiting
Potassium (no U.S. RDA)	all whole foods: meats, milk, fruits, vegetables, grains, legumes	causes muscular weakness, triggers vomiting; if given into a vein, can stop the heart
Sulfur (no U.S. RDA)	all protein-containing foods	would occur only if sulfur amino acids were eaten in excess; this (in animals) depresses growth

The major minerals are calcium, phosphorous, potassium, sulphur, sodium, chloride, and magnesium. These are classified as **macronutrients** because they are found in the body in quantities greater than 100 mg.

The trace minerals, or **micronutrients**, number a dozen or more. The distinction between the major minerals and the trace minerals is one of quantity rather than importance. Deficiencies of either can have serious consequences.

Sodium, potassium, and chloride are the minerals lost primarily through perspiration. Sodium, the positive ion in sodium chloride (table salt), is one of the body's major **electrolytes** (ions that conduct electricity). Americans consume 3 to 4 grams of sodium daily, but the recommendation is to consume only 1.8 to 2.4 grams.[21] Approximately 70 percent of the salt consumed in the United States is in processed foods such as canned and instant soups, smoked meats and fish, cheeses, and deep-fried snacks.

Salt is a cheap preservative and flavor enhancer. The labels on all canned and packaged foods indicate the amount of sodium the product contains. The other 30 percent of our salt intake comes from the salt shaker and from naturally occurring salt in the foods we eat.

Sodium is found in the fluid outside of the cells, and potassium is found within cellular fluid. The temporary exchange of sodium and potassium across the cell's membrane permits the transmission of neural impulses and the contraction of muscles. Low potassium levels interfere with muscle-cell nutrition and lead to muscle weakness and fatigue. Potassium is essential to maintain the heartbeat.

Starvation and very low calorie diets for prolonged periods can lead to sudden death from heart failure as potassium storage drops to critically low levels. Vomiting, diarrhea, and **diuretics** reduce potassium levels. Chronic physical activity that produces heavy sweating probably will not diminish potassium stores unless the diet is woefully lacking in this mineral. It is hard to reduce potassium stores because most foods contain potassium and it is easily replaced. Potassium is particularly abundant in citrus fruits and juices, bananas, dates, nuts, fresh vegetables, meat, and fish.

As with vitamins, mineral intake can be abused. Excessive major and trace minerals produce a variety of symptoms, as shown in Tables 7.7 and 7.8.

Table 7.8   Toxic Symptoms of Trace Minerals

Minerals (U.S. RDA)	Selected Sources	Toxic Symptoms
Iodine (150 g)	iodized salt, seafood	very high intakes depress thyroid activity
Iron (18 mg)	red meats, fish, poultry, shellfish, eggs, legumes, dried fruits	iron overload: infections, liver injury
Zinc (15 mg)	protein-containing foods: meats, fish, poultry, grains, vegetables	fever, nausea, vomiting, diarrhea
Copper (2 mg)	meats, drinking water	unknown except as part of a rare hereditary disease (Wilson's disease)
Fluoride (no U.S. RDA)	drinking water (if naturally fluoride-containing or fluoridated), tea, seafood	fluorosis (discoloration of teeth)
Selenium (no U.S. RDA)	seafood, meat, grains	disorders of digestive system
Chromium (no U.S. RDA)	meats, unrefined foods, fats, vegetable oils	unknown as a nutrition disorder; occupational exposures damage skin and kidneys
Molybdenum, (no U.S. RDA)	legumes, cereals, organ meats	enzyme inhibition
Manganese (no U.S. RDA)	widely distributed in foods	poisoning, nervous system disorders
Cobalt (no U.S. RDA)	meats, milk and milk products	unknown as a nutritional disorder

Water

People can survive for a month or more without food, but a few days without water will result in death. Because all body processes and chemical reactions take place in a liquid medium, the body has to be fully hydrated, and people should make a special effort to replace water when it is lost. Under normal conditions, adults drink 5 to 6 cups of fluid each day. More is needed when the weather is hot and humid and when a person is physically active regardless of weather conditions.

Approximately 60 percent of the body's weight consists of water. Much of it is stored in the muscles, and some is stored in fat. By virtue of his larger muscle mass, the average male stores more water than the average female. Of the total amount of water, 62 percent is found in the intracellular compartment (water within the cells) and the remaining 38 percent is extracellular (water in the blood, lymph system, spinal cord fluid, saliva, and so on).

The water level in the body is maintained primarily by drinking fluids. Solid foods, too, contribute to water replenishment. Many foods—fruits, vegetables, and meats—contain a large percentage of water. Even seemingly dry foods such as bread contain some water. Solid foods add water in another way: They contribute metabolic water, one of the byproducts of their breakdown to energy sources.

Most of the water lost is through urination. Small quantities are lost in feces and in exhaled air from the lungs. Insensible perspiration (that which is not visible) accounts for a considerable amount of water loss. Because exercise and hot, humid weather increase sweating, more water must be consumed during these times. Exercise in hot weather and water replacement guidelines are included in Chapter 6.

The Reduction Equation: Exercise + Sensible Eating = Fat Control

Regular exercise is an important component in weight management. It burns calories, stimulates metabolism, and brings appetite in line with energy expenditure.[22] The two major contributions of exercise are:

1. Preventing overweight/obesity
2. Maintaining post-diet body weight.

The best way to deal with overweight and obesity is to prevent it from occurring in the first place. Second, 95 percent of all dieters who do not exercise during or after the diet regain the lost weight within 3 to 5 years. Researchers at the University of Colorado Health Sciences Center, the University of Pittsburgh School of Medicine, and Brown University examined data from the National Weight Control Registry, which consists of about 3,000 people who have lost a minimum of 30 pounds and maintained the loss for more than one year.[23] These successful dieters were found to have two commonalties: They eat a low-fat diet, and they exercise regularly.

Effects of Exercise on Weight Control

The often neglected factor in a weight-loss attempt is exercise. Exercise and diet are not mutually exclusive. They are complementary in that each has a unique contribution to make to weight loss. The role of exercise was addressed in 1985 at an international meeting on obesity.[24] The unanimous consensus of the experts was that, if you are about to start a weight reduction program or if you are trying to maintain your present weight, success or failure can depend on whether you exercise.

Exercise Burns Calories

The American College of Sports Medicine (ACSM) suggests that the minimal threshold of exercise for weight loss is 300 kcals per exercise session done at least three times a week (900 kcals), or 200 kcals per session performed at least four times a week (800 kcals).[25] These are minimum guidelines. You can turn to Tables 4.2, and 4.3 in Chapter 4, which contain data for walkers and joggers to use to calculate the number of calories expended for a given body weight at a specific speed for a given amount of time.

As fitness improves, the threshold for exercise should increase slowly so the weekly energy expenditure eventually will reach about 2,000 kcals per week. This is considered optimal to enhance health and requires walking or jogging approximately 20 miles per week.

The kcals burned during recovery from exercise contribute marginally to weight loss. The body does not shut off completely after exercise; it recovers gradually. Extra kcals are burned during this period until the metabolism returns to a normal resting level. A rule of thumb is that 15 kcals are burned in recovery for every 100 kcals burned during exercise.[26] If 400 kcals are used during exercise, an extra 60 kcals will be used during the recovery period. Exercising at this level 5 days a week will result in approximately 4½ pounds lost in 1 year from the kcals burned in recovery from exercise. This is illustrated by the following:

$$60 \text{ kcals} \times 5 \text{ days}$$
$$= 300 \text{ kcals/wk} \times 52 \text{ wks}$$
$$= \frac{15,600 \text{ kcals/yr}}{3,500 \text{ kcals}} = 4.45 \text{ lbs}$$

Admittedly, this amount is not much, but it is a bonus that supplements the kcals lost directly through exercise.

Eat More, Weigh Less

Results of animal and human studies during the past 35 years have been equivocal and confusing regarding the effect of exercise on appetite and food intake. The data have shown that exercise decreases, increases, or has no effect upon food intake. Most studies have indicated that people either continued to eat the same amount or increased their food intake when they began exercising and were allowed to eat freely.[27]

In an investigation of the effect of a year of jogging on previously sedentary middle-aged males, the subjects were encouraged not to reduce their food intake or to attempt to lose weight during the course of the study.[28] At the end of one year, the men who ran the most miles had lost the most fat. The more miles they ran, the more they increased their food intake. Those who jogged the most miles (up to 25 miles per week) lost the most fat and the most weight and had the greatest increase in food intake. Many studies have shown that active people consume more kcals, yet are leaner than inactive people.

Two studies at St. Luke's Hospital in New York showed that the effect of exercise on the appetite is regulated to some extent by how obese the person is at the start of the program.[29] After 57 days of moderate treadmill exercise, the obese female subjects had lost an average of 15 pounds. The women's caloric intake during exercise compared to the pre-exercise period was essentially unchanged. This study was repeated with women who were close to ideal weight according to insurance company charts. Moderate treadmill exercise produced an immediate surge in appetite, and the women maintained their "ideal body weight."

Exercise Stimulates Metabolism

Approximately 60 percent to 75 percent of the energy liberated from food is expended to maintain the essential functions of the body.[30] The energy to accomplish these functions is the **basal metabolic rate (BMR)**—the minimum amount of energy that the body expends to sustain life while at complete rest. The BMR is measured at least 12 hours since the last meal, after 8 hours of sleep, and in a thermally neutral environment (at a comfortable room temperature). Because these conditions are difficult to satisfy, they often are approximated, so that the BMR is estimated by the **resting metabolic rate (RMR)**. The RMR requires that measurements be taken 3 to 4 hours after the last meal, following a 30-minute rest period, in a thermally comfortable environment, on a day in which the person has not participated in vigorous physical activity.

Because of less muscle and more fat, the RMR of females is 5 percent to 10 percent lower than males and 15 percent lower than that of very muscular males. Males who are overweight primarily because of heavy musculature have higher RMRs and respond more readily to exercise/diet approaches to weight loss than overweight men whose excess weight is primarily fat.[31] The energy needed to sustain the RMR constitutes a significant amount of the total number of daily calories expended by the average adult. Then, from a weight-management perspective, it is advantageous to preserve or enhance the RMR and to do nothing to reduce it. Exercise fits the bill nicely, particularly resistive exercises that build muscle.

A persistent misconception regarding exercise is that it does not burn enough calories to make the effort worthwhile. Actually, consistent participation in aerobic exercise (such as walking, jogging, cycling, rowing, and aerobic dance) will burn substantial kcals. Anaerobic activities such as weight training do not burn many kcals during the workout, but they build the muscle tissue that will require more kcals later.

Muscle-building activities are an investment in future weight control. In the long run, the increase in muscle mass increases metabolism so the body's kcal requirements increase even at rest. This is why activities for both cardiorespiratory development and muscular development are suggested for weight loss or weight maintenance or, for that matter, any well-rounded physical fitness program.

In the past, the decline in RMR was presumed to be a natural part of aging. But age per se is responsible for only half of the decline while the reduction in physical activity that all too often accompanies aging is responsible for the remainder. **Disuse atrophy**, the loss of muscle tissue from lack of effective stimulation, has a significant negative impact on the RMR because muscle is more metabolically active than fat—it uses more calories than fat under any of life's conditions

Authorities estimate that we lose 3 percent to 5 percent of our active protoplasm (mostly muscle tissue) each decade after 25 years of age.[32] This loss is attributed directly to physical inactivity as we age and results in the all too common negative changes in body composition (an increase in fat and a decrease in lean body mass).

Physical activity is one of the keys to weight management because it uses calories and accelerates metabolism. It also prevents or attenuates the weight-loss plateau that the majority of dieters experience. This plateau represents a period of time when weight loss decelerates substantially or stops temporarily.

For example, young and middle-aged individuals who were within plus or minus 5 percent of their ideal weight, as determined by height, weight, and frame size charts, illustrated the body composition changes that occur with age and physical inactivity.[33] Although both groups were within the ideal range for weight, the middle-aged subjects had twice as much body fat as the young subjects. These data show quite well that lost muscle weight that is replaced by a gain in fat weight produces negative changes in body composition even in the absence of weight gain. Fat is less dense than muscle, so it occupies more room in the body; hence, the change in the configuration of the

Table 7.9 Effects of Physical Inactivity on Body Composition

Subject	Body Weight at Age 20 (lbs)	Body Weight at Age 60 (lbs)	Activity Level	Lean Tissue*	Body Fat	Composition
1	150	150	Inactive	Lost 12%–20%	Gain	Changed
2	150	135	Inactive	Lost 12%–20%	No gain	Changed
3	150	165	Inactive	Lost 12%–20%	Gain	Changed
4	150	150	Active	No Loss	No gain	Unchanged

*The lean tissue values in the table apply to males. The same trend is evident to a lesser extent in females because women have less lean tissue to lose.

Source: Adapted from *Nutrition for Fitness and Sport,* by M. Williams (Dubuque, IA: Wm. C. Brown, 1992).

body. Table 7.9 illustrates some of the changes in body composition that occur as we age. The examples are hypothetical, but they are based upon facts that have been generated over many years of research.

Subject 1 typifies the inactive person who maintains his body weight while aging but undergoes a change in body composition. His bathroom scales provide no clues regarding the change, but the mirror and the fit of his clothes do. This man must hold a tight rein on his appetite because his resting caloric requirements have diminished.

Subject 2 is inactive and chooses to lose weight with age to keep from becoming fatter—rare in U.S. society. He loses one quarter to one half a pound per year after age 30. This individual had lost muscle tissue and has reduced his body weight. His body composition has changed as a result; he is smaller all over. Because of the decline in metabolism from the loss of muscle, along with a lower body weight, which diminishes the caloric cost of any weight-bearing movement, this individual must eat progressively less as the years pass to prevent a gain in fat tissue. Hunger would be a constant companion with this strategy.

Subject 3 probably is most representative of the typical American, who gains both fat and total weight with age. Subject 4 is physically active throughout life. He has little muscle loss and no gain in fat weight. Many examples of this modern-day phenomenon continue to jog, cycle, swim, and so on. Programs that build and maintain muscle tissue preserve the RMR and perpetuate a youthful body composition.

The Effect of Diet on Weight Control

Weight loss attempts in the United States have emphasized dietary restriction with continued sedentary living.[34] This combination has led to consistent failure. Weight loss with this method is temporary, and most of these weight watchers lose and gain weight many times during their life. The eating patterns established during the diet period are short-lived.

People in the United States have been, and continue to be, obsessed with losing weight. At any given time, about 40 percent of women and 25 percent of men are attempting to lose weight for reasons of physical appearance or health.[35] Unfortunately, 90 percent to 95 percent of all dieters regain all or most of the weight that they lost within five years.[36] Eat-less approaches to weight loss and permanent weight control have not worked and probably never will. Inexplicably, people continue to utilize weight-loss strategies that have failed them in the past. New attempts may feature new "diets," but calorie restriction remains the method of choice.

It is time to forget dieting as an effective weight-loss technique. The appropriate nutritional approach emphasizes sensible modifications in eating behavior that can be followed for a lifetime, not for just a few weeks or a few months. This means a nutritional approach that emphasizes a low-fat, high complex-carbohydrate style of eating. This, combined with sensible, progressive, and consistent exercise for a lifetime, should produce the permanent weight loss and control that people want.

Metabolism is affected adversely by calorie restriction.[37] In its quest for **homeostasis** (the tendency to maintain a constancy of internal conditions), the body adapts to the reduced-calorie intake by lowering the metabolic rate. This effort to economize in response to less food intake is a survival mechanism that protects people during lean times. Because the body learns to get by with less, the difference narrows between calories eaten and the calories it needs. This defense mechanism is what has made possible the survival of prisoners of war in concentration camps. Individuals who voluntarily reduce their food intake have the same result: a drop in RMR. As RMR decreases, so, too, does the effectiveness of dieting.

Regular vigorous exercise has the opposite effect: It accelerates the metabolic processes and increases body temperature during and after physical activity. The RMR might remain elevated for some time after exercise. Under exercise conditions, the body is spending kcals rather than hoarding them.

Metabolism represents the body's production of heat. On the one hand, exercise increases heat production, oxygen demand, and calories used. Dieting without exercise, on the other hand, reduces metabolic heat production and, consequently, the number of calories burned. Some studies have shown that several weeks of a very low calorie diet (fewer than 800 kcals/day) resulted in a drop of heat production to 80 percent of the pre-diet level. This is counterproductive because weight loss under this regimen becomes more difficult. As the number of calories needed decreases, the difference between those needed and those consumed becomes smaller. The more restrictive the diet, the greater is the loss of lean tissue and metabolic heat production.

Weight Cycling

Repeated weight loss and regain is referred to as **weight cycling**, also known as cycle dieting and yo-yo dieting. Controversy has arisen regarding the health implications of weight cycling. Some evidence suggests that this practice, if it goes on for a number of years, increases the probability of developing cardiovascular disease. Other evidence shows that weight cycling leads to abdominal fat deposition, greater gains of fat tissue, and a regain of the lost weight plus a few extra pounds than the original amount lost.[38]

All of the above increase the risk for heart disease, stroke, non-insulin-dependent diabetes mellitus, and cancer. Others say a benefit might be associated with weight cycling: When people are in the weight-loss phase of the cycle, their blood pressure and blood fats decrease, along with their risk for Type II diabetes. In short, they are healthier during these periods of lighter body weight. When they regain weight, however, the risks return to pre-diet levels.[39] The surest course of action for overweight and obese people is to lose the weight and keep it off. Figure 7.4 shows the effects of frequent dieting without exercise on body weight.

Waist/Hip Ratio (WHR)

Obesity increases the risk of premature **morbidity** (the sick rate in a population) and **mortality** (the death rate in a population). The distribution of fat is as important as the amount of fat that is deposited. Fat that is distributed regionally in the abdomen, back, and chest—the male pattern, **android obesity**—increases the risk of heart attack, stroke, Type II diabetes, and some forms of cancer.[40] As few as 10 to 15 pounds stored in this manner increases the risk. Fat stored in the hips, buttocks, and thighs—the female pattern, or **gynoid obesity**—is not as risky, but it carries a higher risk than that associated with a normal body weight.

The pattern of fat deposition can be determined by calculating the waist/hip ratio (WHR). Ideally, the hips should be larger than the waist. Use a flexible tape to measure the circumference of your waist at the height of the navel. Then measure your hips at their largest circumference and divide the waist

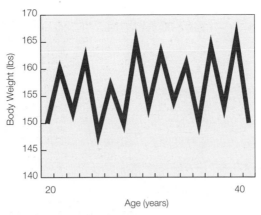

From *Principles and Labs for Fitness and Wellness*, 6th ed. by W. W. K. Hoeger and S. A. Hoeger (Belmont, CA: Wadsworth/Thomson Learning, 2002).

Figure 7.4
Effects of frequent dieting without exercise on body weight.

measurement by the hip measurement. The value obtained can be interpreted as follows:[41]

> **Females:** If the WHR is .8 or greater, the risk is higher than normal.
>
> **Males:** If the WHR is .9 or greater, the risk is higher than normal.

Although the waist/hip ratio is a useful tool, an expert panel convened by the National Heart, Lung, and Blood Institute in 1998 concluded that a waist-circumference measurement alone was equally good or better.[42] The risk for heart disease increases substantially when the waist circumference equals or exceeds 40 inches for males and 35 inches for females. The predictive power of waist circumference is unaffected by height, and its predictive power increases when combined with a body mass index (BMI) greater then 25 Kg/m2. Body mass index is discussed later in this chapter.

Some obese people seem to be diet-resistant. Their weight remains stable even when they are following a low-calorie diet. This irony has been blamed variously upon an underactive thyroid, slow metabolism, or a hereditary tendency toward obesity. A number of studies have shown that the actual reason, in most of these cases, is that the subjects tended to underreport their caloric intake and overestimate their physical activity. This dilemma was examined in a well-controlled study.[43] The researchers found that their diet-resistant subjects underestimated their food intake by 47 percent and overestimated their physical activity by 51 percent. The subjects perceived that their obesity was caused by genetic and metabolic factors rather than errors of judgment regarding caloric consumption and energy expenditure.

The American College of Sports Medicine (ACSM) produced a position paper in 1983, which provided sensible guidelines. With some minor modifications (as identified by statements in brackets below), these are still appropriate today. Some of the important concepts addressed by ACSM are the following:[44]

1. A diet should provide at least 1,200 kcals/day to increase the likelihood of obtaining the necessary nutrients to maintain good health. Diets that are calorically more restrictive are undesirable and potentially dangerous.

2. Food choices should be nutritionally balanced, palatable, and acceptable to the dieter.

3. Weight-loss goals should be moderate—no more than 2 pounds lost per week. [Today some experts support limiting weight loss to 1½ pounds per week.]

4. Behavior modification techniques should be employed in conjunction with dietary modification and exercise to form a well-rounded approach to weight reduction.

5. An endurance-type exercise program is a must. The minimum amount of exercise recommended for weight loss includes participation in exercise 20 to 30 minutes per day, three times per week, at 60 percent of maximum heart rate. [If you expend 300 kcals per exercise session, you can exercise three times per week.]

6. A resistance exercise program [primarily weight training] should accompany the walking or jogging program because it builds the muscle tissue that requires more calories than other bodily tissues, even during rest. The more muscle tissue, the higher is the metabolic rate of burning energy.

7. The dietary modifications and exercise program should be sustainable for a lifetime.

Weight Gain for Underweight People

The focus thus far has been on weight loss rather than weight gain. Nevertheless, the purposeful gain of weight represents a real problem for people who are underweight. What constitutes underweight? This question has not been satisfactorily answered. In any case, actuarial statistics indicate that those who are significantly below the average in body weight have a higher expected mortality rate. Marked underweight can indicate underlying disease and is as much of a risk as obesity for early death.

Being underweight sometimes poses as much of a cosmetic problem for the individual as obesity does for an obese individual. An effective weight-gain program should include regular participation in resistance exercise, in conjunction with three well-balanced meals plus a couple of nutritious snacks between meals. Some commercial drinks are useful for increasing caloric consumption.

Despite herculean efforts, many underweight people find that gaining a pound is more difficult than losing a pound is for the obese.

The amount and type of weight gain should be monitored closely. Gaining muscle tissue without increasing fat stores is desirable. Overeating without exercising will not accomplish this objective, nor will it enhance physical appearance. Body fat should not be increased unless the affected individuals are so thin that they are in danger of dipping into **essential fat**, which is necessary for the life processes.

The key to weight gain is to create a positive energy balance, and the key to muscle weight gain is to effect a positive energy balance, with a higher intake of protein, while participating in a resistive exercise program. Muscle tissue consists of 22 percent protein and 70 percent water, with the remainder being primarily fat and carbohydrate.[45] One pound of muscle tissue contains about 700–800 calories, but it takes the consumption of about 2,500–3,000 extra calories to synthesize that pound. Muscle development is dependent on resistive exercise, a protein intake of 1.5 grams per kilogram of body weight (or .36 grams per pound), and the time (days or weeks) that it takes to consume 2,500–3,000 extra calories.

Measuring Overweight

Overweight is defined as excess weight for one's height. It is assessed by using a height/weight chart or body mass index (BMI). If your weight falls above the acceptable range, you are overweight. This approach does not make allowances for body composition. It just provides information about weight status without taking into account the person's fluid, fat, or muscle make-up. Two people of the same sex, same height, and same weight conceivably could differ considerably in physical appearance because one might be carrying excess fat while the other is carrying substantial muscle tissue. Besides the difference in physical appearance, the risk of developing premature chronic disease is associated with excess fat, not muscle.

A method for assessing overweight that is popular with medical and nutrition researchers is the **body mass index (BMI)**. Some authorities consider it to be the best available method for assessing **percent body fat**.[46] Its inherent limitation—because it is based on height and weight—is similar to that of the height/weight tables. Muscular people can fall into the overweight category without being overfat. Advantages of this method are:

- the ease with which it can be determined
- the establishment of BMI categories that identify weight status
- the identification of BMI levels that constitute a risk for cardiovascular disease.

Body mass index can be determined easily from Table 7.10 by reading the directions at the top of the table. If your weight falls between two columns, however, you will have to extrapolate. For example, a person who is 68 inches tall and weighs 163 pounds is half the distance between 158 lbs and 164 pounds, which translates into half the distance between 24 and 25 Kg/M², or 24.5 KgM². Table 7.11 provides an interpretation of BMI values.[47]

Measuring Body Composition

Body composition assessment requires the separation and quantification of lean tissue from fat. Many indirect methods for measuring this component have been developed but we will focus on just one—**skinfold** measurements.

Lean tissue includes all tissue except fat: muscle, bones, organs, fluid, and the like. Fat includes both essential and storage fat. Essential fat, found in the bone marrow, organs, muscles, intestines, and central nervous system, is indispensable to normal physiological functioning.

The amount of essential fat in the male body is equal to approximately 3 percent to 5 percent of the total body weight. The amount of essential fat in

Table 7.10   Body Mass Index Table BMI (kg/m²)

Directions: Each entry gives the body weight in pounds for a person of a given height and BMI. Pounds have been rounded to the nearest whole number. Find your height in the far left column and move horizontally across the row to your body weight. The number at the top of the column is your BMI.

Height (Inches)	19	20	21	22	23	24	25	26	27	28	29	30	35	40
						Body Weight (Pounds)								
58	91	96	100	105	110	115	119	124	129	134	138	143	167	191
59	94	99	104	109	114	119	124	128	133	138	143	148	173	198
60	97	102	107	112	118	123	128	133	138	143	148	153	179	204
61	100	106	111	116	122	127	132	137	143	148	153	158	185	211
62	104	109	115	120	126	131	136	142	147	153	158	164	191	218
63	107	113	118	124	130	135	141	146	152	158	163	169	197	225
64	110	116	122	128	134	140	145	151	157	163	169	174	204	232
65	114	120	126	132	138	144	150	156	162	168	174	180	210	240
66	118	124	130	136	142	148	155	161	167	173	179	186	216	247
67	121	127	134	140	146	153	159	166	172	178	185	191	223	255
68	125	131	138	144	151	158	164	171	177	184	190	197	230	262
69	128	135	142	149	155	162	169	176	182	189	196	203	236	270
70	132	139	146	153	160	167	174	181	188	195	202	207	243	278
71	136	143	150	157	165	172	179	186	193	200	208	215	230	286
72	140	147	154	162	169	177	184	191	199	296	213	221	258	294
73	144	151	159	166	174	182	189	197	204	212	219	227	265	302
74	148	155	163	171	179	186	194	202	210	218	225	233	272	311
75	152	160	168	176	184	192	200	208	216	224	232	240	279	319
76	156	164	172	180	189	197	205	213	221	230	238	246	287	328

Table 7.11   Guidelines for Interpreting BMI

Classification	Grade	BMI Kg/m²
1. Underweight		<18.5
2. Acceptable		18.5–24.9
3. Overweight		25–29.9
4. Obesity	I	30–34.9
	II	35–39.9
5. Extreme Obesity	III	≥40

These values are the same for both sexes.
< less than
≥ equal to or greater than

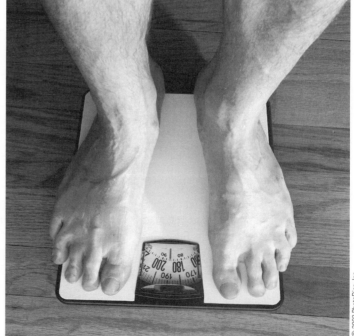

Body weight is not an indicator of body fat.

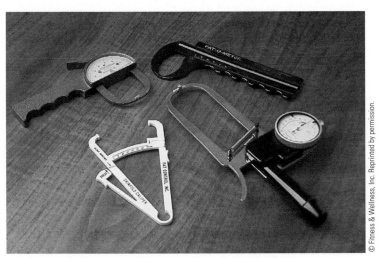

Various types of calipers are used to assess skinfold thickness.

the female body is equal to about 11 percent to 14 percent of the total body weight. The disparity in the amount of essential fat between the sexes is probably because of sex-specific essential fat stored in a female's breasts, pelvic area, and thighs. Essential fat constitutes a lower limit beyond which fat loss is undesirable and unhealthy because of the possibility of impaired normal physiological and biological functioning from such loss.

Storage fat is found in **adipose** (fat) tissue. For most people, this represents a substantial energy reserve. Adipose cells are found subcutaneously (under the skin) and around the organs, where they act as a buffer against physical trauma. Reducing excess storage fat is desirable for health and aesthetic reasons. Reasonable goals for total body fat (essential plus storage fat) differ by sex. Excellent values for males and females are 12 percent and 20 percent, respectively. Males are **overfat** when 25 percent or more of their weight is in the form of fat. Females are overfat when 32 percent or more of their weight is in the form of fat.[48]

Skinfold measurement became more common after several low-cost calipers made their way into the marketplace. In skilled hands, some of them correlate quite well (.90) with the more expensive brands found in most exercise physiology labs.

The rationale for the skinfold technique is that approximately half of the body's fat is located directly beneath the skin. Therefore, the skinfold—which consists of a double layer of skin and the underlying fat—can be measured using a caliper. Tables for age and sex are used to convert skinfold measurement (in millimeters) to percent fat. These are given in Tables 7.12 and 7.13.

To become proficient, the person administering the skinfold test practices measuring the different sites for all ages and both sexes. The method can be standardized by observing the following suggestions:

1. Mark each site according to the directions given in Figure 7.5.
2. Take two measurements at each site, unless the two differ by more than 1 millimeter. In that case, take a third measurement and average the two closest readings.
3. Apply the calipers about 1/4 inch to 1/2 inch below the fingers. This allows the calipers rather than the fingers to compress the skinfold.
4. Ensure that the calipers maintain contact with the skinfold for 2 to 5 seconds so the reading can stabilize.

Table 7.12   Percent Fat Estimates For Men*

Sum of Skinfolds (mm)	Age to the Last Year								
	Under 22	23 to 27	28 to 32	33 to 37	38 to 42	43 to 47	48 to 52	53 to 57	Over 57
8– 10	1.3	1.8	2.3	2.9	3.4	3.9	4.5	5.0	5.5
11– 13	2.2	2.8	3.3	3.9	4.4	4.9	5.5	6.0	6.5
14– 16	3.2	3.8	4.3	4.8	5.4	5.9	6.4	7.0	7.5
17– 19	4.2	4.7	5.3	5.8	6.3	6.9	7.4	8.0	8.5
20– 22	5.1	5.7	6.2	6.8	7.3	7.9	8.4	8.9	9.5
23– 25	6.1	6.6	7.2	7.7	8.3	8.8	9.4	9.9	10.5
26– 28	7.0	7.6	8.1	8.7	9.2	9.8	10.3	10.9	11.4
29– 31	8.0	8.5	9.1	9.6	10.2	10.7	11.3	11.8	12.4
32– 34	8.9	9.4	10.0	10.5	11.5	11.6	12.2	12.8	13.3
35– 37	9.8	10.4	10.9	11.5	12.0	12.6	13.1	13.7	14.3
38– 40	10.7	11.3	11.8	12.4	12.9	13.5	14.1	14.6	15.2
41– 43	11.6	12.2	12.7	13.3	13.8	14.4	15.0	15.5	16.1
44– 46	12.5	13.1	13.6	14.2	14.7	15.3	15.9	16.4	17.0
47– 49	13.4	13.9	14.5	15.1	15.6	16.2	16.8	17.3	17.9
50– 52	14.3	14.8	15.4	15.9	16.5	17.1	17.6	18.2	18.8
53– 55	15.1	15.7	16.2	16.8	17.4	17.9	18.5	19.1	19.7
56– 58	16.0	16.5	17.1	17.7	18.2	18.8	19.4	20.0	20.5
59– 61	16.9	17.4	17.9	18.5	19.1	19.7	20.2	20.8	21.4
62– 64	17.6	18.2	18.8	19.4	19.9	20.5	21.1	21.7	22.2
65– 67	18.5	19.0	19.6	20.2	20.8	21.3	21.9	22.5	23.1
68– 70	19.3	19.9	20.4	21.0	21.6	22.2	22.7	23.3	23.9
71– 73	20.1	20.7	21.2	21.8	22.4	23.0	23.6	24.1	24.7
74– 76	20.9	21.5	22.0	22.6	23.2	23.8	24.4	25.0	25.5
77– 79	21.7	22.2	22.8	23.4	24.0	24.6	25.2	25.8	26.3
80– 82	22.4	23.0	23.6	24.2	24.8	25.4	25.9	26.5	27.1
83– 85	23.2	23.8	24.4	25.0	25.5	26.1	26.7	27.3	27.9
86– 88	24.0	24.5	25.1	25.7	26.3	26.9	27.5	28.1	28.7
89– 91	24.7	25.3	25.9	26.5	27.1	27.6	28.2	28.8	29.4
92– 94	25.4	26.0	26.6	27.2	27.8	28.4	29.0	29.6	30.2
95– 97	26.1	26.7	27.3	27.9	28.5	29.1	29.7	30.3	30.9
98–100	26.9	27.4	28.0	28.6	29.2	29.8	30.4	31.0	31.6
101–103	27.5	28.1	28.7	29.3	29.9	30.5	31.1	31.7	32.3
104–106	28.2	28.8	29.4	30.0	30.6	31.2	31.8	32.4	33.0
107–109	28.9	29.5	30.1	30.7	31.3	31.9	32.5	33.1	33.7
110–112	29.6	30.2	30.8	31.4	32.0	32.6	33.2	33.8	34.4
113–115	30.2	30.8	31.4	32.0	32.6	33.2	33.8	34.5	35.1
116–118	30.9	31.5	32.1	32.7	33.3	33.9	34.5	35.1	35.7
119–121	31.5	32.1	32.7	33.3	33.9	34.5	35.1	35.7	36.4
122–124	32.1	32.7	33.3	33.9	34.5	35.1	35.8	36.4	37.0
125–127	32.7	33.3	33.9	34.5	35.1	35.8	36.4	37.0	37.6

*Sum of chest, abdominal, and thigh skinfolds.

"Practical Assessment of Body Composition," by A. S. Jackson and M. L. Pollock, *The Physician and Sportsmedicine*, 13:5 (1985), 76–90. Reprinted by permission.

Table 7.13   Percent Fat Estimates For Women*

Sum of Skinfolds (mm)	Under 22	23 to 27	28 to 32	33 to 37	38 to 42	43 to 47	48 to 52	53 to 57	Over 57
					Age to the Last Year				
23– 25	9.7	9.9	10.2	10.4	10.7	10.9	11.2	11.4	11.7
26– 28	11.0	11.2	11.5	11.7	12.0	12.3	12.5	12.7	13.0
29– 31	12.3	12.5	12.8	13.0	13.3	13.5	13.8	14.0	14.3
32– 34	13.6	13.8	14.0	14.3	14.5	14.8	15.0	15.3	15.5
35– 37	14.8	15.0	15.3	15.5	15.8	16.0	16.3	16.5	16.8
38– 40	16.0	16.3	16.5	16.7	17.0	17.2	17.5	17.7	18.0
41– 43	17.2	17.4	17.7	17.9	18.2	18.4	18.7	18.9	19.2
44– 46	18.3	18.6	18.8	19.1	19.3	19.6	19.8	20.1	20.3
47– 49	19.5	19.7	20.0	20.2	20.5	20.7	21.0	21.2	21.5
50– 52	20.6	20.8	21.1	21.3	21.6	21.8	22.1	22.3	22.6
53– 55	21.7	21.9	22.1	22.4	22.6	22.9	23.1	23.4	23.6
56– 58	22.7	23.0	23.2	23.4	23.7	23.9	24.2	24.4	24.7
59– 61	23.7	24.0	24.2	24.5	24.7	25.0	25.2	25.5	25.7
62– 64	24.7	25.0	25.2	25.5	25.7	26.0	26.2	26.4	26.7
65– 67	25.7	25.9	26.2	26.4	26.7	26.9	27.2	27.4	27.7
68– 70	26.6	26.9	27.1	27.4	27.6	27.9	28.1	28.4	28.6
71– 73	27.5	27.8	28.0	28.3	28.5	28.8	29.0	29.3	29.5
74– 76	28.4	28.8	28.9	29.2	29.4	29.7	29.9	30.2	30.4
77– 79	29.3	29.5	29.8	30.0	30.3	30.5	30.8	31.0	31.3
80– 82	30.1	30.4	30.6	30.9	31.1	31.4	31.6	31.9	32.1
83– 85	30.9	31.2	31.4	31.7	31.9	32.2	32.4	32.7	32.9
86– 88	31.7	32.0	32.2	32.5	32.7	32.9	33.2	33.4	33.7
89– 91	32.5	32.7	33.0	33.2	33.5	33.7	33.9	34.2	34.4
92– 94	33.2	33.4	33.7	33.9	34.2	34.4	34.7	34.9	35.2
95– 97	33.9	34.1	34.4	34.6	34.9	35.1	35.4	35.6	35.9
98–100	34.6	34.8	35.1	35.3	35.5	35.8	36.0	36.3	36.5
101–103	35.3	35.4	35.7	35.9	36.2	36.4	36.7	36.9	37.2
104–106	35.8	36.1	36.3	36.6	36.8	37.1	37.3	37.5	37.8
107–109	36.4	36.7	36.9	37.1	37.4	37.6	37.9	38.1	38.4
110–112	37.0	37.2	37.5	37.7	38.0	38.2	38.5	38.7	38.9
113–115	37.5	37.8	38.0	38.2	38.5	38.7	39.0	39.2	39.5
116–118	38.0	38.3	38.5	38.8	39.0	39.3	39.5	39.7	40.0
119–121	38.5	38.7	39.0	39.2	39.5	39.7	40.0	40.2	40.5
122–124	39.0	39.2	39.4	39.7	39.9	40.2	40.4	40.7	40.9
125–127	39.4	39.6	39.9	40.0	40.4	40.6	40.9	41.1	41.4
128–130	39.8	40.0	40.3	40.5	40.8	41.0	41.3	41.5	41.8

*Sum of triceps, suprailium, and thigh skinfolds.

"Practical Assessment of Body Composition," by A. S. Jackson and M. L. Pollock, *The Physician and Sportsmedicine*, 13:5 (1985), 76–90. Reprinted by permission.

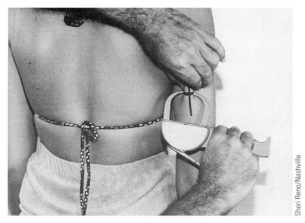

Triceps Skinfold. Take a vertical fold on the midline of the upper arm over the triceps halfway between the acromion and olecranon processes (tip of shoulder to tip of elbow). The arm should be extended and relaxed when the measurement is taken.

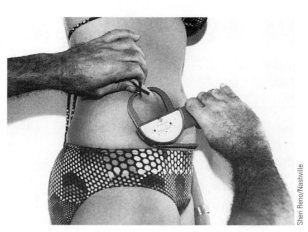

Suprailium Skinfold. Take a diagonal fold above the crest of the ilium directly below the mid-axilla (armpit).

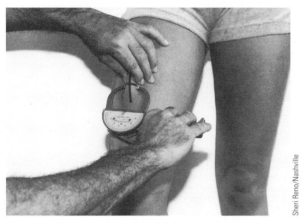

Thigh Skinfold. Take a vertical fold on the front of the thigh midway between the hip and knee joint.

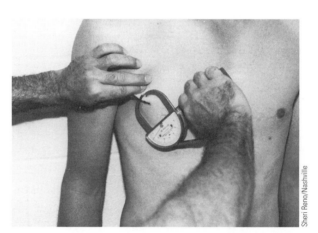

Chest Skinfold. Take a diagonal fold one-half the distance between the anterior axillary line and nipple.

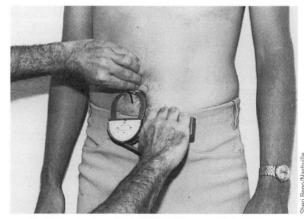

Abdominal Skinfold. Take a vertical fold about 3/8 inch from the navel.

Figure 7.5 Skinfold measurement sites.

Terms

Adipose	Macronutrients
Amino acids	Micronutrients
Anabolism	Morbidity
Android obesity	Mortality
Antioxidants	Nutrient-dense
Basal metabolic rate (BMR)	Nutrients
	Overfat
Body mass index (BMI)	Overweight
	Oxidation
Carcinogenic	Percent body fat
Catabolism	Percent daily value
Dietary Reference Intake (DRI)	Phytochemicals
	Phytoestrogens
DNA	Phytomedicinals
Disuse atrophy	Resting metabolic rate (RMR)
Diuretics	
Electrolytes	Skinfold
Essential fat	Soluble fiber
Free radicals	Storage fat
Gynoid obesity	Transfatty acids
Homeostasis	Triglycerides
Hydrogenation	Waist/hip ratio (WHR)
Insoluble fiber	
Lipids	Weight cycling

Summary

- ❖ Metabolism is the sum total of chemical reactions whereby the energy liberated from food is made available to the body. It consists of two processes—anabolism and catabolism.

- ❖ The Food Guide Pyramid has replaced the basic four food group as the primary guidelines for food choices.

- ❖ The food labels mandated by the federal government for processed food give quantities of various nutrients and caloric values that help consumers make more informed food choices.

- ❖ Carbohydrates consist of simple sugars and starches.

- ❖ Sugar causes tooth decay but is not an independent risk factor for chronic diseases except in rare cases.

- ❖ Sugar consumption continues to rise in the United States.

- ❖ Fiber is an indigestible polysaccharide that is beneficial to health. The two types of dietary fiber are soluble and insoluble.

- ❖ Carbohydrates yield 4 kcals/gram.

- ❖ Fats are energy-dense, yielding 9 kcals/gram.

- ❖ Saturated fats come from animal flesh, dairy products, and tropical oils. This type of fat raises serum cholesterol levels.

- ❖ Unsaturated fats come from plants and should constitute the majority of the fat we consume.

- ❖ Dietary fat should be less than 30 percent of the total caloric intake.

- ❖ Transfatty acids could be as harmful as saturated fats. This artificial fat (made through the process of hydrogenation) makes up 5 percent to 10 percent of the fat in the average U. S. diet.

- ❖ Protein intake should be about 15 percent of the total calories consumed.

- ❖ Adults need .8 of a gram of protein per kg of body weight; endurance athletes require about twice this amount.

- ❖ The fat-soluble vitamins are A, D, E, and K; the water-soluble vitamins are C and B complex.

- ❖ Antioxidant vitamins are thought to play an important role in preventing cardiovascular disease and cancer.

- ❖ Free radicals are harmful body products that damage cells; they can be contained by consuming abundance of antioxidant vitamins, found in vegetables and fruits.

- ❖ Minerals are inorganic substances that the body requires; they are classified as major minerals or trace minerals.

- ❖ Exercise is an important component of weight management because it burns calories and stimulates metabolism. Dieters decrease their caloric intake but, without exercise, reduce their metabolism and lean body tissue instead of fat.

❖ Most dieters regain the lost weight within 5 years.

❖ Weight cycling (yo-yo dieting) increases the risk for cardiovascular disease.

❖ Being underweight may be a health hazard as well as a cosmetic problem for some people.

❖ To gain weight, the underweight should eat three nutritious meals and a couple of between-meal snacks plus participate in a sound weight training program.

❖ Android obesity (male) increases the risk of heart attack, stroke, type II diabetes, and some forms of cancer. Gynoid obesity (female) likewise increases the risk for "lifestyle diseases."

❖ Body mass index (BMI) is a good method for determining one's weight status.

❖ Males have less essential fat than females.

❖ Skinfold measurement techniques are inexpensive, quick, and effective for measuring percent body fat.

Notes

1. Editors, "Special Report: Portion Distortion," *Tufts University Health and Nutrition Letter*, 18:12 (Feb. 2001), 4–5.

2. Editors, "Healthy Behaviors Achieved by Few," *Fitness Management Magazine*, 17:12 (Nov. 2001), 16.

3. H. M. Ali, B.A. Bowman, E. S. Ford, et al, "The Continuing Epidemics of Obesity and Diabetes in the United States," *Journal of the American Medical Association*, 286:10 (Sept. 12, 2001), pp. 1579–1581.

4. U. S. Department of Health and Human Services, *Healthy People 2010*, 2d ed.: *With Understanding and Improving Health and Objectives for Improving Health* (2 vols.). (Washington, DC: U. S. Government Printing Office, 2000).

5. B. L. Marks, "Tobacco Exposure and Chronic Illness," *ACSM's Resource Manual,* edited by J. L. Roitman (Philadelphia: Lippincott Williams and Wilkins, 2001).

6. B. S. Worthington-Roberts and S. R. Williams, Editors *Nutrition Throughout the Life Cycle* (Boston: McGraw Hill, 2000).

7. S. Margen and the Editors, "Wellness Nutrition Counter," University of California at Berkeley *Wellness Letter* (New York: Rebus, 1997).

8. B. Liebman, "Sugar: The Sweetening of the American Diet," *Nutrition Action Health Letter*, 25:9 (Nov. 1998), 1–7.

9. M. Jacobson, "Liquid Candy," *Nutrition Action Health Letter*, 25:9 (Nov. 1998), 8.

10. Editors, "Is Sugar Bad for You?" *Harvard Health Letter*, 26:4 (2001), 1–2.

11. J. Dahl, "Sugars and Fats: The Tip of the Food Pyramid," *Cardi Sense*, 4:2 (1994), 6.

12. U. S. Department of Health and Human Services, *Nutrition and Your Health: Dietary Guidelines for Americans* (Washington, DC: U. S. Government Printing Office, 2000).

13. Editors, "Should You be Choosing Foods by Their Glycemic Index?" *Tufts University Health and Nutrition Letter*, 18:9 (Nov. 2000), 4–5.

14. Editors, Consumer Union, "Fish: Weighing The Risks and Benefits," *Consumer Reports On Health*, 13:4 (2001), 1, 4.

15. T. Byers, "Hardened Fats, Hardened Arteries?" *New England Journal of Medicine*, 337:21 (Nov. 20, 1997), 1554–1545.

16. Editors, "Chewing the Fats: AHA Conference Prompts New Look at Monos, Polys, and Trans," *Environmental Nutrition*, 23:7 (2000) 1, 6; S. Poindexter, L. St. Clair, and K. Wheeler, "Diet and Chronic Disease," *ACSM's Resource Manual*, edited by J. L. Roitman (Philadelphia: Lippincott Williams and Wilkins, 2001).

17. Editors, "Trans Fatty Acids Expected to Appear on Nutrition Facts Labels," *Tufts University Health and Nutrition Letter*, 17:12 (2000), 3.

18. G. M. Wardlaw, *Contemporary Nutrition* (Boston: McGraw Hill Higher Education, 2000).

19. Wardlaw, Note 18.

20. B. N. Ames, M. K. Shigenaga, and T. M. Hagen, "Oxidants, Antioxidants, and the Degenerative Diseases of Aging," *Proceedings of the National Academy of Sciences*, 90 (1993), 7915–7922.

21. S. Margolis and L. B. Wilder, *Nutrition and Longevity* (Baltimore: Johns Hopkins Medical Institutions, 1999).

22. C. M. Grillo and K. D. Brownell, "Intervention for Weight Management," *ACSM's Resource Manual,* edited by J. L. Roitman (Philadelphia: Lippincott Williams and Wilkins, 2001).

23. Editors, "High-Protein Diets: When Lost Pounds Come Back to Haunt You," *Tufts*

University Health and Nutrition Letter, 19:3 (May 2001), 1.

24. W. R. Foster and B. T. Burton (eds), "Health Implications of Obesity: National Institutes of Health Development Conference," *Annals of Internal Medicine,* 103:977, Supplement 6, Part 2, 1985.

25. ACSM, *Guidelines for Exercise Testing and Prescription* (Philadelphia: Lippincott Williams and Wilkins, 2000).

26. D. C. Nieman, *Exercise Testing and Prescription: A Health-Related Approach* (Mountain View, CA: Mayfield, 1999).

27. Grillo and Brownell, Note 22.

28. P. D. Wood et al., "Increased Exercise Level and Plasma Lipoprotein Concentrations: A One-Year Randomized, Controlled Study in Sedentary Middle-Aged Men," *Metabolism,* 32 (1983), 31.

29. P. Wood, *California Diet and Exercise Program* (Mountain View, CA: Anderson World Books, 1983).

30. D. C. Nieman, *Exercise Testing and Prescription A Health-Related Approach* (Mountain View, CA: Mayfield, 1999).

31. C. Pierre, "Maximizing Metabolism: Can Calorie Burning be Increased?" *Environmental Nutrition,* 12 (Feb. 1989), 1.

32. R. A. Robergs and S. O. Roberts, *Exercise Physiology for Fitness, Performance, and Health* (Boston: McGraw Hill Higher Education, 2000).

33. M. H. Williams, *Lifetime Fitness and Wellness* (Madison, WI: Brown and Benchmark, 1996).

34. "Losing Weight: A New Attitude Emerges," *Harvard Heart Letter,* 4:7 (March 1994), 1.

35. "Heavy News," University of California at Berkeley *Wellness Letter,* 10:5 (Feb. 1994), 2.

36. S. Margolis and L. J. Cheskin, *Weight Control* (New York: Medletter Associates, 1998).

37. Nieman, Note 30.

38. Wardlaw, Note 18.

39. Wardlaw, Note 18.

40. J. P. Despres, "Visceral Obesity, Insulin Resistance, and Dyslipidemia: Contribution of Endurance Exercise Training to the Treatment of Plurimetabolic Syndrome," *Exercise and Sport Sciences Reviews,* 25 (1997), 271–300.

41. D. Isreal, "Nutrition," *ACSM's Resource Manual,* edited by J. L. Roitman (Philadelphia: Lippincott Williams and Wilkins, 2001).

42. NHLBI Obesity Education Initiative Expert Panel, *Clinical Guidelines on the Identification, Evaluation and Treatment of Overweight and Obesity in Adults* (Washington, DC: National Heart, Lung, and Blood Institute, 1998).

43. S. W. Lichtman et al., "Discrepancy between Self-Reported and Actual Caloric Intake and Exercise in Obese Subjects," *New England Journal of Medicine,* 327 (1992), 1893.

44. American College of Sports Medicine. "Proper and Improper Weight Loss Programs," *Medicine and Science in Sports and Exercise,* 15 (1983), ix.

45. Williams, Note 33.

46. NHLBI, Note 42.

47. "Guidelines Call More Americans Overweight," *Harvard Health Letter,* 23:10 (Aug. 1998), 7.

48. S. K. Powers and E. T. Howley, *Exercise Physiology Theory and Application to Fitness and Performance* (Boston: McGraw Hill Higher Education, 2001).

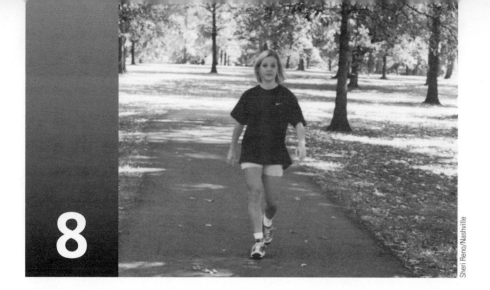

Sheri Reno/Nashville

Reducing the Risk of Selected Diseases Through Exercise

Outline

The health benefits associated with walking and jogging, as well as other aerobic exercises, have been researched systematically during the last couple of decades. Evidence supporting health enhancement through consistent participation in physical exercise has been accumulating steadily. This chapter focuses on the effect of exercise in preventing, delaying, and, to a lesser extent, treating coronary heart disease and other selected diseases.

Cardiovascular Diseases

Cardiovascular diseases—diseases of the heart and blood vessels—comprise the leading causes of death in the United States. They are responsible for approximately 39 percent of the total number of deaths annually.[1] In the United States, 58,000,000 people have one or more forms of cardiovascular disease, nearly 1 million of whom die each year.[2]

The leading form of cardiovascular disease, claiming nearly 500,000 lives annually, is **coronary heart disease**.[3] This is the classic disease that leads to heart attack when obstructions (blood clots) or spasms (constricture

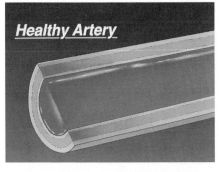
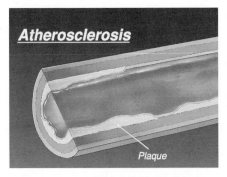
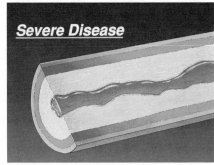

Figure 8.1 Plaque build-up at various stages of atherosclerosis.

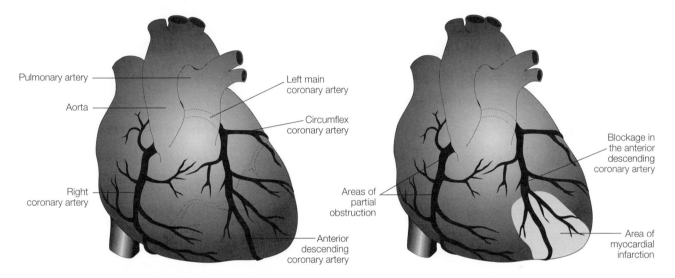

Figure 8.2 Heart attack caused by blood clot.

of coronary vessels) disrupt the flow of blood to a portion of the heart muscle. The site of obstruction or spasm determines the extent of muscle damage.

Heart attacks of any magnitude result in irreversible injury and death of the heart muscle. The dead muscle forms scar tissue that no longer contributes to the heart's ability to pump blood. After a heart attack, the heart becomes a less efficient pump. If the attack is massive and causes extensive damage, the heart and its host will die.

The primary cause of coronary heart disease is **atherosclerosis**, a condition in which fatty substances, cholesterol, calcium, fibrin, and cellular debris form plaques over time that obstruct the flow of blood. If unchecked, plaques continue to enlarge until the arterial channels narrow significantly, creating the environment for blood clots or spasms at these sites. If blood flow is completely impeded, a heart attack will occur and muscle tissue damage will follow (see Figures 8.1 and 8.2).

Risk Factors for Heart Disease

Although most heart attacks occur later in the life cycle (55 percent after 65 years of age), the processes responsible begin quite early, often before adolescence. Atherosclerosis is responsible for about 80 percent of all heart attacks. It is the result of interactions between genetic factors and lifestyle behaviors.

Certain lifestyle behaviors were identified by the Framingham Heart Disease Study as risk factors for coronary heart disease. The risks are generally categorized as those that can be changed and those that cannot. Major risk factors that cannot be changed are increasing age, male gender, and heredity.

Age

The statistical probability that a person will die from heart disease increases with advancing age. In fact, 55 percent of all heart attacks occur after 65 years of age, and 85 percent of all fatal heart attacks occur after 65 years of age.

Male Gender

Men are, and have been, the primary candidates for heart disease. An alarming trend has surfaced in recent years though: **Morbidity** (the sick rate in a population) and **mortality** (the death rate in a population) have been increasing steadily in premenopausal women. The prime contributor is cigarette smoking, and when it is coupled with taking oral contraceptives, the risk increases substantially.

Coronary heart disease is the leading cause of death and disability among women, accounting for almost 235,000 deaths annually.[4] By age 65, a woman's risk is approximately the same as a man of the same age.[5] On average, women tend to get heart disease about 10 years later than men, so men are at higher risk at younger ages. But the risk equals out and eventually reverses at and beyond 65 years of age.[6]

Prior to **menopause** (permanent stoppage of the menstrual cycle) women are at less risk than men because estrogen, the female sex hormone, protects the coronary arteries from premature disease. Also, women have a more favorable blood–fat ratio that protects the arteries from athero-sclerosis. Vulnerability to heart disease for women increases after menopause because estrogen production decreases and then stops, and blood–fat ratios change so they resemble the masculine profile.

Heredity

Children whose parents have heart disease or atherosclerosis have an increased tendency to develop these problems themselves. A family history of heart disease is confirmed when (a) a father or first-degree male relative (grandfather or brother) has had a clinically diagnosed heart attack or dies of heart disease prior to 55 years of age, and (b) a mother or first-degree female relative (grandmother or sister) has had a clinically diagnosed heart attack or dies of heart disease prior to 65 years of age.[7] Having a family history increases an individual's estimated risk by approximately 25 percent, which is about one-tenth as dangerous as cigarette smoking.[8] This is not intended to imply that a positive family history is insignificant but, rather, that its effect should not be overestimated.

Other risk factors can be changed. These include cigarette smoking, high blood pressure, elevated serum cholesterol, physical inactivity, obesity, diabetes, and individuals' responses to stress.

Cigarette Smoking

Many medical researchers consider cigarette smoking to be the most potent of the preventable risk factors associated with chronic illness and premature death. It is directly responsible for 419,000 deaths from all causes in the United States. Smoking accounts for 30 percent of all deaths from cancer and 30 percent of all cardiovascular deaths.[9]

Tobacco smoke contains more than 4,000 chemicals, 60 of which are **carcinogenic** (capable of producing cancer).[10] Two of the most noxious of these are nicotine and carbon monoxide.

Nicotine is an addictive, stimulant drug that releases chemicals that raise the heart rate, blood pressure, and resting and physical-activity metabolism. Carbon monoxide, the same gas that is emitted from the exhaust of automobiles, trucks, and buses, is a poisonous gas that competes with oxygen for binding sites on hemoglobin.

Hemoglobin (a protein pigment transported by red blood cells that attaches to and carries oxygen) has a much greater affinity for carbon monoxide than it has for oxygen. As a result, there is a proportional decrease in oxygen that is displaced by carbon monoxide. This is a significant problem that is further complicated by the fact that carbon monoxide has a half-life of 5½ hours after it attaches to hemoglobin. By comparison, oxygen detaches from hemoglobin in just a matter of minutes.

An increased level of carbon monoxide combined with nicotine act in concert to reduce HDL-cholesterol, to increase blood platelet adhesiveness (which increases the likelihood of arterial spasms), to increase fibrinogen (which increases the probability of clot formation), and increases levels of homocysteine (a protein that increases the risk of having a heart attack). These factors, individually or together, predispose people prematurely to coronary heart disease. The answer is: Stop smoking or, better yet, don't start.

Passive Smoke and Smokeless Tobacco Products

Passive smoke (also called involuntary, secondhand, or environmental smoking) involves inhaling the smoke of others. Those who breathe secondhand smoke have increased risk of premature illness and death. Estimates show that 35,000 to 60,000 nonsmokers die annually of heart disease because of exposure to secondhand smoke, and another 3,000 die of lung cancer.[11]

Inhaling secondhand smoke has a dose-response relationship with developing smoking-related illnesses. The greater the exposure, the greater is the risk. Children of smoking parents have a higher incidence of influenza, bronchitis, asthma, pneumonia, and the common cold.

In recent years smokeless tobacco products (chews, plugs, and dips) have become increasingly popular with high school and college males. These products pose another threat. Nicotine is just as addictive and just as harmful when it is delivered through the oral cavity as it is when delivered through the lungs. The effects of carbon monoxide are eliminated from smokeless tobacco products because these are not combustible, but users of smokeless tobacco trade less risk of lung cancer for greater risk of oral cancer. The incidence of oral cancer is 50 times higher among users than among nonusers.[12]

Tobacco use is an extremely difficult habit to break. Success requires overcoming the addiction to nicotine while simultaneously dealing with the psychological dependence. The latter might be more of a challenge than the former. The person overcomes the nicotine addiction within the first couple of weeks after quitting, but the psychological and social cues remain for years. Breaking this dependence requires reeducation and changes in behavior.

Stop-smoking approaches include professional counseling, nicotine patches, nicotine chewing gum, hypnosis, artificial cigarettes, acupuncture, and aversive conditioning. The 1-year success rates for these techniques range from 10 percent to 40 percent. Millions of Americans have quit smoking. The number of adult smokers today is half that of the 1960s.

Exercise offers another option. When people get hooked on the exercise habit, they often disconnect from the smoking habit. Smoking is a drawback to exercise performance, and it limits the health gains that can be achieved with exercise.

High Blood Pressure

Blood pressure is recorded in millimeters of mercury (mmHg). It is the combined force that circulating blood exerts against the artery walls plus the resistance to blood flow by the arteries. Pressure is created as the heart contracts and pumps blood into the arteries. The smallest arteries (the arterioles) offer resistance to blood flow. If the resistance is consistently high, the pressure increases and remains high. The medical term for high blood pressure is **hypertension.**

Hypertension has no overt symptoms. It is a silent disease that can be detected only by a blood pressure screening test. Blood pressure consists of two components:

1. **Systolic pressure** represents the maximum pressure of blood flow in the arteries when the heart contracts.

2. **Diastolic pressure** represents the minimum pressure of blood flow in the arteries between heartbeats.

Blood pressure is read as the systolic over the diastolic pressure. A reading of 140/90 or greater is considered to be hypertensive. A blood pressure of 100/60 is considered to be the lowest level of normal; however, some people with lower values function normally and are free of disease. A low normal reading is highly desirable. Table 8.1 classifies blood pressure from normal to hypertension.

Approximately 50 million Americans have blood pressure above 140/90. The causes of 90 percent to 95 percent of these cases are unknown. This type of hypertension is called "essential," which is a medical term that means "of unknown origin or cause." Although **essential hypertension** cannot be cured, it can be treated and, usually, controlled.

Longstanding uncontrolled or poorly controlled hypertension has an adverse effect on the heart. High blood pressure increases the heart's workload, and the heart enlarges in response to the strain. Because the blood pressure is consistently high, the heart does not get enough rest. As a result, the heart's muscle fibers become overstretched and progressively lose their ability to rebound. The end result is that the force of contraction weakens and the heart becomes an inefficient pump. If intervention strategies are not enacted early in the process, the heart will suffer irreversible damage. Hypertension also has a detrimental effect on the arteries and accelerates the atherosclerotic process.

Prevention techniques include maintaining recommended body weight, restricting dietary salt, ingesting adequate calcium and potassium, engaging in voluntary relaxation, and exercising regularly. Aerobic exercises such as walking and jogging help to control blood pressure.

Based on the evidence, the American College of Sports Medicine (ACSM) has taken the position that "endurance (aerobic) exercise training by individuals at high risk for developing hypertension will reduce the rise in blood pressure that occurs with time."[13] Furthermore, aerobic exercises performed at moderate intensity (40 percent to 70 percent of aerobic capacity) seem to lower blood pressure as much as, and sometimes more than, exercises performed at higher intensities. Moderately intense aerobic exercises performed three to five days per week for 20 to 60 minutes per workout lower both systolic and diastolic pressure by 10 mmHg.[14]

How does aerobic exercise lower blood pressure? *First*, the hormones epinephrine and norepinephrine play

Table 8.1   Standards for Classification of Blood Pressure for Adults Age 18 Years and Older

Category	Systolic (mmHg)	Diastolic (mmHg)
Normal	< 130	< 85
High Normal	130–139	85–89
Hypertension		
Stage 1 (Mild)	140–159	90–99
Stage 2 (Moderate)	160–179	100–109
Stage 3 (Severe)	180–209	110–119
Stage 4 (Very Severe)	≥ 210	≥ 120

From National Institutes of Health, *The Fifth Report of the Joint National Committee on Detection, Evaluation and Treatment of High Blood Pressure* (Washington, DC: U.S. Dept. of Health and Human Services, January, 1993) NIH Publication No. 93–1088.

important roles in regulating blood pressure. Both are **vasoconstrictors** —they clamp down on the **arterioles**, which requires more force to circulate blood through them. Aerobic training decreases the circulating levels of these hormones, which allows the arterioles to relax and widen. Exercise keeps the arteries limber. This response lowers the resistance to blood flow, which in turn lowers the blood pressure.[15]

Second, aerobic exercise increases cells' sensitivity to **insulin,** a hormone that facilitates the passage of sugar from the blood to the cells. Sugar (glucose) is an important source of energy that the cells use to perform their normal functions. Increased sensitivity to insulin yields an important bonus: The kidneys excrete excess sodium, and this also lowers the blood pressure. *Third*, aerobic exercise contributes to weight loss, which lowers the blood pressure.[16]

High Serum Cholesterol

Cholesterol is a steroid required for the manufacture of hormones and bile (for the digestion and absorption of fats); it is one of the structural components of neural tissue; and it is required for the construction of cell walls. Although a certain amount of cholesterol is needed for good health, an excessive amount in the blood— **serum cholesterol**—is associated with heart attacks and strokes.

Strokes, or "brain attacks," are a result of blood clots blocking the flow of blood to portions of the brain or a hemorrhage in the brain resulting from a blood vessel that has burst (see Figure 8.3). Common consequences of a stroke are paralysis of one side of the body and slurred speech. If a stroke is massive, the victim dies.

People obtain cholesterol in two ways:

1. External, through dietary consumption

2. Internal, by the body manufacturing its own.

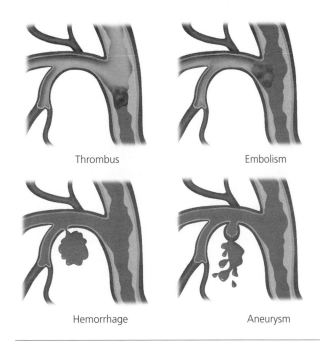

Thrombus   Embolism

Hemorrhage   Aneurysm

Figure 8.3 Causes of a stroke.

NHLBI Guidelines

New recommendations for detecting and lowering blood cholesterol were released by the National Heart, Lung, and Blood Institute (NHLBI) in May 2001. Table 8.2 illustrates the new categories of risk. The NHLBI also urged physicians to pay closer attention to a cluster of factors that substantially contribute to the development of heart disease. These factors, collectively referred to the **metabolic syndrome,** include excessive abdominal fat, high blood pressure, high blood sugar, elevated triglycerides, and low HDL cholesterol.[17]

The new guidelines also state that the maximum daily consumption of cholesterol should be reduced from less than 300 mg/day to less than 200 mg/day; saturated fat intake should be lowered from less than 8 percent of the total calories to less than 7 percent; and total fat intake may be increased from 30 percent to 35 percent of the total daily calories, provided that the majority of these come from monounsaturated and polyunsaturated sources. The guidelines stress the importance of maintaining a normal body weight and consistent participation in physical exercise.

Table 8.2 Risk Profile—Lipid and Lipoprotein Concentrations

Total Cholesterol	Category of Risk
1. < 200 mg/dL[a]	Desirable
2. 200–239 mg/dL	Borderline high
3. ≥ 240 mg/dL[b]	High

LDL Cholesterol	Category of Risk
1. < 100 mg/dL	Optimal
2. 100–129 mg/dL	Near optimal/above optimal
3. 130–159 mg/dL	Borderline high
4. 160–189 mg/dL	High
5. ≥ 190 mg/dL	Very high

HDL Cholesterol	Category of Risk
1. ≤ 40 mg/dL[c]	Increased risk
2. ≥ 60 mg/dL	Heart protective

Triglycerides	Category of Risk
1. < 150 mg/dL	Normal
2. 150–199 mg/dL	Borderline high
3. 200–499 mg/dL	High
4. ≥ 500 mg/dL	Very high

a. < is less than
b. ≥ is equal to or greater than
c. ≤ is equal to or less than

Adapted from "Revised Cholesterol Guidelines," *Harvard Heart Letter*, 11:11 (July 2001), 6–7.

We have made significant progress in reducing our dietary cholesterol over the last three decades, but we need no dietary intake of cholesterol because the liver manufactures all of the cholesterol the body needs.

Saturated fat is the primary ingredient from which cholesterol is produced inside the body. As a result, most authorities are more concerned about the amount of saturated fat than cholesterol we consume—but they are quick to add that it is prudent to limit the intake of both.

Dietary cholesterol and saturated fat are found in animal flesh, eggs, whole milk, and whole-milk dairy products. Fruits and vegetables are free of cholesterol, and—with a few exceptions—also are low in fat. Coconuts, coconut oil, palm oil, and palm kernel oil are high in saturated fat. Olives, nuts and seeds, and avocados are high in monounsaturated fat, which is a less harmful form.

The amount of cholesterol circulating in the blood is expressed in milligrams per deciliter (mg/dL), so a cholesterol level of 210 is read as 210 mg/dL. Table 8.2 indicates levels of risk for total serum cholesterol.

Maintaining a desirable value of serum cholesterol reduces the risk. For every 1 percent that serum cholesterol is lowered, the risk of heart disease is reduced by 2 percent to 3 percent.[18]

Cholesterol Carriers

Knowing one's total serum cholesterol value tells only part of the story. To fully evaluate the cholesterol risk, we must know our total cholesterol (TC) as well as two of its important fractions —the low density lipoprotein (LDL) fraction and the high density lipoprotein (HDL) fraction. The **lipoproteins** are carriers to which cholesterol attaches for transport through the circulatory system.

LDL cholesterol is the most atherogenic (capable of developing atherosclerosis) of all of the cholesterol sub-fractions. But LDLs become dangerous only when their numbers are excessive and are accompanied by the advancement of lesions (injuries) to the artery walls. As a result, LDLs are able to infiltrate the artery, where they become toxic and initiate a series of bodily responses that lead to the development of atherosclerosis.

LDL cholesterol can be lowered through weight loss if overweight, reduction in dietary intake of fat and cholesterol, increase in dietary fiber and soy protein, exercise, and medication if needed.[19] Table 8.2 presents the relative risks associated with LDL cholesterol.

HDL—high density lipoproteins— protect the arteries from atherosclerosis because they act as scavengers that collect cholesterol from other lipoproteins, and probably from arterial plaque, and shuttle it back to the liver, where it is degraded and removed from the body. A low number of circulating HDLs is a powerful predictor of heart disease. Table 8.2 illustrates HDL values and their relative risk.

Aerobic exercises such as walking, jogging, cycling, and stair-stepping, performed at a moderate to vigorous level, increase HDLs by about 20 percent.[20] Other strategies for increasing HDLs include weight loss if overweight, low-dose alcohol consumption, avoidance of tobacco smoke, and reduction in dietary simple sugars.[21]

Alcohol also can be a substance of abuse. Overuse or misuse contributes to 100,000 deaths annually in the United States.[22]

In addition to raising HDLs, low-dose alcohol (up to 1.5 ounces of alcohol per day for females and 3 ounces per day for males) acts as an anti-inflammatory and it keeps the blood platelets from clumping together thereby inhibiting clot formation. But this must be weighed against the fact that even low dose alcohol is harmful to all of the body's cells, tissues, and organs. Non drinkers should not start drinking on their own. A physician should decide whether to prescribe low dose alcohol based on the patient's history and current status of risk factors.

Determining Cholesterol Risk

An accurate assessment of cholesterol risk requires measurement of total cholesterol (TC) and the LDL and HDL fractions. A desirable total cholesterol still can put one at significant risk if the LDLs are too high or the HDLs are too low. The cardiac risk can be evaluated by the "cholesterol ratio" when the results of cholesterol testing are contradictory, such as when HDLs and LDLs are both high or both low.[23] The cholesterol ratio is calculated by dividing total cholesterol by HDL cholesterol, and the result can be interpreted by referring to Table 8.3.

Triglycerides

Triglycerides are one of the body's major sources of fuel for muscular movement. These fats are obtained through the consumption of dietary fats, and they also are produced by the liver from carbohydrates. Triglycerides are necessary for good health, but high levels are harmful (see Table 8.2). Research has indicated that

Table 8.3   Ratio of Total Cholesterol to HDL

Risk	Male	Female
Very Low (½ of average)	<3.4*	<3.3
Low	4.0	3.8
Average	5.0	4.5
Moderate (2 × average)	9.5	7.0
High (3 × average)	>23**	>11.0

* < less than
** > greater than

elevated triglycerides are a modest independent risk factor for heart disease but, when coupled with low HDLs, the risk increases substantially.[24]

Triglycerides can be lowered by losing weight; reducing dietary intake of saturated fat, cholesterol, simple sugars, and alcohol; eating more fiber-rich foods, fruits, and vegetables; eating one or two fish meals per week; and exercising regularly.

Physical Inactivity

Physical inactivity is debilitating to the human body. Humans illustrate the biological dictate, "Use it or lose it." That which we use becomes stronger, while that which we do not use becomes weaker. All body systems and all muscles, including the heart muscle, respond to this principle.

The results of a number of important investigations have concluded that physical inactivity is a major risk for heart disease. Those who exercise consistently, even at low intensity, tend to be healthier and to live longer than people who are sedentary. The ongoing Harvard Alumni Study found that the minimum exercise threshold for increasing longevity was as little as walking 5 miles per week.[25] Those who walked or jogged 20 to 22 miles per week achieved optimal benefits. They lived an average of 2 years longer than sedentary people.

Investigators at the Cooper Institute for Aerobics Research found that physically fit subjects who had high blood pressure or elevated serum cholesterol were less likely to die prematurely from all causes than unfit individuals with normal values of both.[26] The Centers for Disease Control and Prevention concluded that exercise is the one lifestyle change that could most affect health status.[27] This is based primarily on the fact that more than 60 percent of Americans are either sedentary or they exercise too infrequently to enhance their health.

Health enhancement through physical activity does not require a great deal of effort. The requirement is 30 minutes of physical activity at least 4 days per week every week. There are few constraints on the type of activities that can be chosen. All physical activities (including cycling, jogging, walking, and swimming, among many others), most games and sports, many leisure-time activities, and some occupational work have the potential to meet the minimum criteria for improving health. Exercise, in sum, has the following cardiovascular benefits:

1. Increases HDL-cholesterol

2. Decreases LDL-cholesterol

3. Favorably changes the ratios between total cholesterol and HDL, and between LDL and HDL-cholesterol

4. Decreases triglyceride levels

5. Promotes relaxation; relieves stress and tension

6. Decreases body fat and favorably changes body composition

7. Reduces blood pressure, especially if it is high

8. Makes blood platelets less sticky

9. Results in fewer cardiac arrhythmias

10. Increases myocardial efficiency
    a. Lowers resting heart rate
    b. Increases stroke volume

11. Increases oxygen-carrying capacity of the blood

Exercise on a regular basis has been emphasized in this text because it is the *only* way to improve fitness and health simultaneously. Another important reason for consistent participation in exercise is that it reduces the risk of sudden death from a heart attack during and immediately after sporadic physical exertion (such as shoveling snow).

Two studies, one completed in the United States and the other in Germany, documented this observation. The U. S. study showed that sedentary people were 100 times more vulnerable to incurring a heart attack during strenuous activity than at other times.[28] In contrast, those who exercise consistently face only a small increase in the risk, but the health and fitness benefits from training far outweigh the minimal risk.[29]

Obesity

The current perception of obesity is that it is a chronic disease like hypertension or diabetes rather than a simple failure of willpower. Data indicate that Americans once again are gaining weight. The number of overweight males has risen from 24 percent to 32 percent, and the number of overweight females has risen from 27 percent to 35 percent.[30]

Excess body weight carries medical consequences. Obesity increases the risk and the consequences of many other chronic diseases. It significantly increases the workload of the heart, and it coexists with high blood pressure and elevated serum cholesterol. Obesity is related to the onset of diabetes, arthritis, and some forms of cancer. Estimates indicate that obesity is involved in 300,000 premature deaths from all causes each year.[31]

The National Institutes of Health define **obesity** as 20 percent above desirable weight. Other authorities define it relative to the percent of body weight that consists of fat. This is a more accurate method that provides guidelines for weight loss and weight control. Males are obese when 25 percent or more of their total body weight is in the form of fat. Females are obese when 32 percent or more of their total body weight is in the form of fat.

Excessive fat is a risk, and the manner in which it is distributed also has to be considered. Abdominal fat increases the risk for heart attacks, stroke, diabetes, and some forms of cancer. Even as few as 15 extra pounds stored in this pattern increases the risk substantially. A waist circumference of 35 inches or greater for females or 40 inches or greater for males increases the risk for coronary heart disease, and the predictability for heart disease increases when these measurements are coupled with a body mass index of 25 kg/m² or more.[32] Fat that is stored in the hips, buttocks, and thighs presents less of a risk.

Fortunately, obesity is reversible. When the excess weight is lost, the risk subsides. Weight loss strategies are discussed in Chapter 7.

Diabetes Mellitus

Diabetes mellitus is a metabolic disorder in which the body is unable to regulate the level of blood glucose (sugar). It is one of the 10 leading causes of death in the United States. Diabetics who die prematurely succumb to complications of the disease. These include cardiovascular lesions, accelerated atherosclerosis, and heart disease. Diabetics also are susceptible to kidney disease, nerve and blood vessel damage, blindness, and lower-limb amputation resulting from gangrene. In addition, diabetes tends to elevate the serum cholesterol and creates an environment in the circulatory system that facilitates the development of blood clots. Diabetes is a major risk for coronary heart disease.[33]

The two types of diabetes mellitus are:

1. *Type I*—usually occurring early in life. Victims of Type I diabetes don't produce insulin, so they must take it by daily injection. Without insulin, sugar would accumulate in the blood and spill out of the body through the kidneys. The body would be forced to use fat as its primary fuel, producing serious consequences for the diabetic person. Although diabetes cannot be cured, it can be controlled. Living a well-regulated life that includes exercise, weight control, and a low-fat diet is paramount to controlling Type I diabetes.

2. *Type II*—occurring about middle age, to overweight, underactive people. This form of diabetes may or may not require medication. Lifestyle factors are important in treating and controlling Type II diabetes. Many authorities predict that at least 75 percent of all cases of Type II diabetes could be prevented by maintaining normal body weight and by exercising regularly.[34]

A landmark piece of research, *The Physician's Health Study*, showed that exercise reduced the risk of developing Type II diabetes.[35] Type II accounts for 90 percent of all cases of diabetes. Physicians who exercised vigorously five or more times per week had a 42 percent reduction in the incidence of Type II diabetes compared to those who exercised less than once a week. Each 500 calories burned per week in physical activity reduces the risk of Type II diabetes by 6 percent.[36] The reduction in the risk was particularly evident in those at greatest risk—the obese. The researchers concluded that at least 24 percent of all Type II diabetes was related to a sedentary lifestyle.

Stress

Although stress is difficult to quantify, authorities tend to agree that chronic stress or distress produces physiological changes in the body that can predispose people to illness. Stress also hastens the process of **subclinical disease**.

Chronic stress can have a detrimental effect on the immune system for months or years. Stress stimulates the secretion of above normal amounts of hormones, collectively called the **catecholamines**, that circulate at high levels in the bloodstream. The catecholamines rev up the body's engine so it runs at high throttle. Physical exercise is the antidote because it metabolizes these products and thereby lowers their level in the

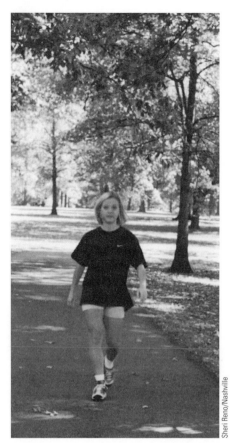

Regular moderate exercises—such as walking—strengthen the immune system.

blood. But the catecholamine level of sedentary people remains elevated so the arterioles are in a constant state of slight contraction. This condition, known as **peripheral vascular resistance**, increases the workload of the heart.

Situations and circumstances are stressful only if we allow them to be. The stressor is not what produces the problem. It is the way we perceive and react to it. Two people confronted by the same stressor might exhibit different reactions. For example, delivering a speech to a group of people is anxiety-producing and threatening to one of them and is an exciting challenge to another. We cannot avoid stress. It is part of life in our competitive, dynamic society.

Among the stressful events we might have to deal with are divorce, death of a loved one, layoff from a job, and retirement. Because we cannot avoid stress, we must learn to manage it. Exercise is a beneficial coping mechanism that rids the body of stress-initiated harmful products that accumulate over time.

New and Emerging Risk Factors

Research has increased our knowledge of risk factors for cardiovascular disease. Two advances relate to homocysteine and another form of lipoprotein.

Homocysteine

Homocysteine is one of the amino-acid-building blocks of protein. It is carried in the blood, and under normal conditions it splits into two other amino acids. When it does not split, homocysteine blood levels rise, increasing the risk for heart disease.

High homocysteine levels damage the inner lining of the arteries.[37] The lesions, or injuries, that it causes stimulate the abnormal growth of smooth muscle cells in the artery walls, which in turn promote the development and progression of atherosclerosis. Homocysteine levels can be controlled through proper diet. The B vitamins **folic acid** (folate), B_6, and B_{12} are needed to process homocysteine.

Lipoprotein (a)

Lipoprotein (a) represents a group of particles that resemble low density lipoprotein (LDL-C). Many scientists believe that high levels of **Lp(a)** promote the development of blood clots in the arteries. In addition, they enhance the plaque-forming ability of LDL-C. Lp(a) levels are determined primarily by genetic make-up. Lifestyle behaviors that lower the risk for coronary heart disease seem to have no effect when it comes to lowering Lp(a).[38] Therefore, people with high blood levels of Lp(a) should concentrate on lowering risk factors over which they have control, such as total cholesterol and its sub-fractions, blood pressure, body weight, and tobacco use. Equally important is a regular exercise program.

Cancer

Cancer, the second leading cause of death in the U. S., is responsible for one in every four deaths.[39] Projected estimates for 2001 indicated that 553,400 people would die from cancer and 1,268,000 new cases would be diagnosed. Lung cancer is the leading cause of cancer deaths for both men and women. The second leading cause of cancer deaths for men and women, respectively, are prostate and breast cancer.[40]

Cancer is actually a general term that applies to more than 100 diseases characterized by abnormal and uncontrolled cellular growth. Any cell can become cancerous if it is exposed under conducive conditions to carcinogenic (cancer-producing) substances. Exposure to carcinogens eventually will give rise to mutant cells, which will divide and grow uncontrollably. Normal cells follow an orderly and predictable blueprint for growth and division. Cancerous cells do not respond to the body's signals restricting cellular division, so they and their offspring continue to grow wildly. The mass of new growth is a tumor or **neoplasm** (new tissue).

Cancerous tumors are **malignant**. They grow rapidly, and they are not confined or localized. They shed their cells, invade surrounding tissues, and compete with normal cells for space and nutrients. **Metastasis** is the medical term for the spread of cancer from its original site to other areas of the body. The processes that transform normal cells to malignant ones are complex and not well understood.

Techniques and strategies have emerged that can reduce the incidence of many forms of cancer. Cancer prevention includes:

1. Abstinence from all forms of tobacco

2. A diet rich in fruits, vegetables, and grains, low in fat, and devoid of smoked and cured meat and fish

3. Minimum exposure to radiation and carcinogenic chemicals such as asbestos and radon gas

4. Regular participation in exercise

5. Maintenance of normal body weight throughout life.

An international panel of cancer experts has concluded that 30 percent to 40 percent of all cancer cases worldwide could be prevented by consuming a healthy diet, getting regular exercise, and maintaining an appropriate body weight.[41] Many studies have shown that the most physically active people have the least risk of developing cancer. Men whose cardiorespiratory fitness was low had almost double the risk of dying from cancer as those who were most fit.[42]

The strongest evidence for a protective effect of exercise exists for colon, breast, and prostate cancers.[43] Aerobic exercises such as walking and jogging that are performed at a moderate to vigorous intensity may reduce

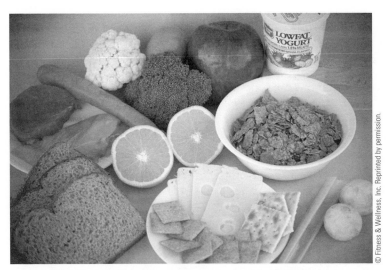

Fruits, vegetables, and grains contribute to a healthy anti-cancer diet.

the risk for these and possibly other forms of cancer by:

1. Preventing weight gain and obesity

2. Strengthening the immune system

3. Speeding the transit time of food through the intestines, resulting in less time for contact between fecal matter and the intestinal walls.

4. Reducing the production of estrogen in females, lowering the risk for breast cancer, and testosterone in males, lowering the risk for prostate cancer.

Osteoporosis

Osteoporosis is a silent chronic disease that produces a loss of bone mass resulting in structural deterioration of the skeleton and increased susceptibility to bone breakage. Building and maintaining bone density is a lifetime pursuit.[44] The bones reach peak density between the ages of 20 and 30, but 90 percent of adult bone mineral content is deposited by the end of adolescence.[45] This is a time when youngsters of both sexes should be getting enough calcium (approximately 1,200 to 1,500 mg/day), vitamin D (400 IU/day), and consistent exercise of a weight-bearing aerobic type plus weight training.

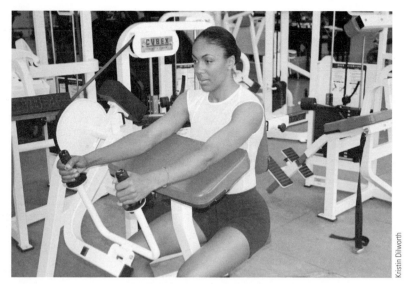

Kristin Dilworth

Resistance exercises protect the skeletal system from osteoporosis.

The most common fracture sites associated with osteoporosis are vertebral crush fractures (bones of the spinal column) and fractures of the hip, wrist, and femur (thigh bone). The death rate within the first year after a hip fracture in an elderly person is 18 percent to 33 percent, and most of those who survive have a diminished quality of life.[46]

Risk Factors for Osteoporosis

Some factors that increase the likelihood of developing osteoporosis are:

1. *Age*
2. *Gender.* Women are more susceptible than men, particularly those with a small, thin skeletal framework and those who experience early menopause. Men also develop osteoporosis, but they lose bone more slowly and usually incur bone fractures when they are older.
3. *Heredity.* The risk is greater when other family members have osteoporosis.
4. *Lack of physical activity.* Physical activity stresses the bones and maintains the integrity of the skeletal system.
5. *Cigarette smoking:* Smoking suppresses estrogen production in

females, leading to early menopause and loss of the skeletal protection provided by estrogen.

6. *Insufficient intake of calcium and vitamin D.* It is probably effective and prudent to suggest that all adults consume 1,200 to 1,500 mg of calcium from food and supplements each day. Vitamin D is needed for the body to absorb calcium. Adults up to 60 years of age should take in 400 IU (International Unit) of vitamin D daily; adults ages 60 to 69 should increase to 600 IU daily; and those ages 70 and older should take in 800 IU daily.

Although osteoporosis is treatable, it is not curable. The best approach is to prevent or delay its advent. The most important preventive technique is to develop as much bone as possible during the teenage years.

Effects of Exercise

Bone is living tissue that responds to the downward force of gravity and the lateral forces generated by the forceful contraction of muscles. Weight-bearing, impact-loading exercises such as walking, jogging, aerobic dancing, and stair-climbing can increase bone mass.[47] Even the skeletal systems of nursing-home residents (average age 87 years) have responded to exercise with an increase in bone mass. Non-weight-bearing activities such as swimming and stationary cycling are not as effective in increasing bone density.[48]

Researchers have examined the effect of resistance weight training on the skeletal system. Studies have indicated that bones respond to weight training by becoming thicker and denser.[49] For good results, weight-training exercises should be done at an intensity level equal to 80 percent of 1 repetition maximum (1RM). This is approximately equivalent to performing 10 lifts, or repetitions, of an exercise with a weight heavy enough so it cannot be lifted 11 times. Exercises that stress the major muscle groups should be selected so the bones to which they are attached also will be stressed.

Osteoarthritis

Osteoarthritis is the most common of the many forms of arthritis. Osteoarthritis leads to decline of the soft, smooth cartilage at the surface of joints. This happens to some people as early as 30 years of age. Osteoarthritis causes minimal inflammation of the affected joints.

A myth that seems to persist is that jogging causes premature osteoarthritis of the knees. This perception is fueled by the biomechanics of jogging, which indicates that the force developed at the knee when the foot strikes the ground is six times that of the force generated by walking. As a result, many have concluded that jogging must be harmful to the knees.

Contradicting that conclusion, 35 years of data collection and analysis by researchers in the Framingham Heart Study indicated that the major cause of osteoarthritis of the knees is obesity.[50] In fact, high-mileage running—an average of 28 miles per week for a minimum of 12 years—was not associated with the premature development of osteoarthritis.

A later study confirmed the Framingham conclusion. This investigation found that persons in the upper 20 percent of body weight experienced 7 to 10 times the risk of developing osteoarthritis of the knees and hips than those whose body weight was in the lowest 20 percent.[51]

Individuals with osteoarthritis need to exercise because it increases strength, promotes flexibility, reduces pain, controls body weight, preserves mobility, and enhances well-being.[52] The health of cartilage, which has no blood supply of its own, depends on regular stimulation and use of the joints. When the joints move, fluid and waste products are squeezed out of cartilage. When the joint relaxes, fluid seeps back in, bringing oxygen and nutrients with it. Rhythmic contractions of the muscles lubricate and nourish the joints.

If osteoarthritis is present already, impact-loading exercises could aggravate the condition and produce pain. If this happens, a simple shift to low-impact non-weight-bearing exercises should bring relief and allow continued participation. Appropriate activities include walking, water walking, water aerobics, and swimming. Other acceptable activities include the use of stationary cycles, rowing machines, and cross-country ski machines.

Asthma

The American Thoracic Society has defined asthma as the increased responsiveness of the trachea (windpipe) and bronchi (the two main subdivisions of the trachea that transport air to and from the lungs) to a variety of stimuli resulting in airway obstruction that is reversible spontaneously or as a result of treatment. Breathing becomes difficult during an asthma attack, and this can be frightening.

In the United States, 14 million people are asthmatic and more than 5,000 die from asthma-related conditions each year.[53] Asthma affects about 5 percent of all Americans.[54] Although asthma has no cure, medications are available to effectively prevent or reduce the length and severity of an attack.

Asthmatics often remain sedentary because of their fear of exercise-induced asthma (EIA). But asthma should not deter children, adolescents, and older adults from participating in physical activities. The American Academy of Allergy and Immunology encourages regular exercise for asthmatics, who receive the same health benefits as other individuals. People with asthma have competed successfully in sports at national and international levels.

Asthmatics who want to exercise or who currently are exercising can use the same method of prevention that Olympic athletes practice.

1. Airway-opening drugs should be used immediately prior to exercise or competition.

2. A gradual warm-up period of 15 minutes should be followed by a 15-minute period of rest. This protocol reduces the probability of incurring exercise-induced asthma for about 2 hours.

3. Treatment must be individualized to find the optimal regimen for each individual. This will involve several trial-and-error attempts before determining the best approach.

The types and intensity of exercise that contribute to the onset of exercise-induced asthma have been identified. The mechanisms responsible for EIA are the loss of respiratory heat and water because of the high rate of breathing during exercise. The more intense the exercise, the greater is the loss of heat and water. Therefore, the more intense forms of exercise usually are the most **asthmogenic** (capable of inducing bronchospasms).

Swimming and other water activities are the least asthmogenic types of exercise. This is probably attributable primarily to the warm, moist environment in which they are done and, second, because the high breathing rates necessary to initiate bronchospasms are difficult to achieve.[55] Running and cycling seem to be the most asthmogenic of the outdoor activities, but the risk can be minimized by following the guidelines for Olympic athletes alluded to earlier.

Depression

Clinical depression is prolonged sadness that persists for some time. It is characterized by depressed mood and loss of interest in all activities for a minimum of 2 weeks.[56] These behaviors are accompanied by at least four of the following symptoms:

1. Change in appetite

2. Sleep disturbance

3. Fatigue

4. Feelings of guilt or worthlessness

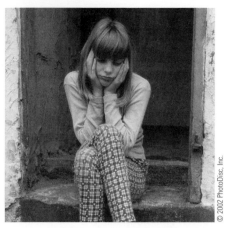

Depression can range from a mild form of blues to severe clinical depression.

5. Difficulty concentrating

6. Suicidal thoughts.

Exercise is one component in the spectrum of treatments for depression.[57] Studies have shown that aerobic exercises, primarily walking and jogging, have improved the mental health status of depressed patients. Many of these patients improved dramatically enough to be taken off medication, and the improvement of others led to a reduction in medications. The patients who exercised the most improved the most.

Terms

Arterioles	LDL
Asthmogenic	Lipoproteins
Atherosclerosis	Lp(a)
Cardiovascular	Malignant
diseases	Menopause
Carcinogenic	Metabolic
Catecholamines	syndrome
Clinical depression	Metastasis
Coronary heart	Morbidity
disease	Mortality
Diastolic pressure	Neoplasm
Essential	Obesity
hypertension	Peripheral vascular
Folic acid	resistance
HDL	Serum cholesterol
Hemoglobin	Subclinical disease
Homocysteine	Systolic pressure
Hypertension	Vasoconstrictors
Insulin	

Summary

❖ The leading form of cardiovascular disease—claiming about half a million lives annually—is coronary heart disease.

❖ Coronary heart disease is characterized by obstructions (blood clots or spasms) in the coronary arteries that lead to a reduction or stoppage of blood flow to portions of the heart muscle.

❖ Atherosclerosis is a slow, progressive disease of large and mid-size arteries that is responsible for about 80 percent of all heart attacks.

❖ Risk factors are genetic or learned behaviors that increase the probability of premature illness and death from a specific chronic disease.

❖ The statistical probability that death will result from heart disease increases with advancing age.

❖ Women contract heart disease about 10 years later than men, but the risk equals out and eventually reverses at and beyond the age of 65.

❖ Children whose parents have heart disease or atherosclerosis have an increased tendency to develop these conditions.

❖ Cigarette smoking is responsible for nearly a third of mortality from heart disease.

❖ Nicotine is a powerful addictive stimulant that has profound adverse effect on the cardiovascular system.

❖ The carbon monoxide in cigarette smoke displaces oxygen and reduces the oxygen-carrying capacity of the blood.

❖ Breathing secondhand smoke is harmful to nonsmokers.

❖ Smokeless tobacco products are addictive and harmful.

❖ High blood pressure, or hypertension, adversely affects the heart and its blood vessels.

❖ Essential hypertension is the most common form of high blood pressure.

❖ Lifestyle behaviors that can prevent or treat hypertension include exercise, weight loss, salt restriction, optimum calcium and potassium intake, and voluntary relaxation techniques.

❖ Cholesterol is found in animal flesh, eggs, whole milk, and whole-milk dairy products.

❖ The liver manufactures cholesterol from fats, including saturated fat.

❖ Dietary intake of cholesterol is unnecessary because the liver manufactures all of the cholesterol the body needs.

❖ The NHLBI issued new guidelines for detecting and treating cholesterol.

❖ LDL cholesterol is implicated in the development of atherosclerosis.

❖ LDLs are dangerous when their numbers are excessive and lesions occur to the artery walls.

❖ HDL cholesterol protects the arteries by removing cholesterol from the blood.

❖ People who exercise consistently tend to be healthier and live longer than people who are sedentary, and their HDL cholesterol is usually higher.

❖ High levels of triglycerides are a modest risk factor for heart disease.

❖ The risk of sudden death during and immediately after exercise is much more likely in unfit people.

❖ The number of overweight people has increased notably.

❖ Obesity is considered a disease and is a risk factor for other chronic diseases as well.

❖ The android pattern of fat deposition increases the risk of heart disease, stroke, diabetes, and some forms of cancer.

❖ Diabetes mellitus is a metabolic disorder in which the body is unable to regulate the level of blood glucose.

❖ Type I diabetes usually appears early in life and requires the daily injection of insulin.

❖ Type II diabetes usually arises about middle-age to overweight and underexercised people. The Physician's Health Study concluded that at least 24 percent of all Type II diabetes is related to a sedentary lifestyle.

❖ Stress suppresses the immune system. Because we cannot avoid stress, we must learn to manage it.

❖ Homocysteine in the blood damages the arteries and increases the risk for heart attack.

❖ Lp(a) increases the likelihood of developing blood clots and forming plaque in the arteries.

❖ Cancer is the second leading cause of death in the United States.

❖ Lung cancer is the leading cause of deaths from cancer for men and women alike.

❖ Cancer is characterized by abnormal and uncontrollable cellular growth.

❖ Thirty to forty percent of all cancer cases worldwide could be prevented by consuming a healthy diet, getting regular exercise, and maintaining an appropriate body weight.

❖ Exercise helps to prevent cancer by reducing body fat, stimulating the immune system, and increasing the transit of food through the digestive system.

❖ Osteoporosis is a "silent" disease characterized by the gradual loss of bone mass.

❖ Women are affected by osteoporosis more often and at an earlier age than men.

❖ Risk factors for osteoporosis include age, gender, heredity, lack of physical activity, cigarette smoking, and insufficient calcium intake.

❖ Osteoporosis is treatable but not curable.

❖ Weight-bearing aerobic exercises and weight-training exercise are best for developing and maintaining the skeletal system.

❖ Osteoarthritis is the result of wear of the cartilage between joints.

❖ The major cause of osteoarthritis is obesity.

❖ Exercise alleviates osteoarthritis by lubricating and nourishing the joints.

❖ Nonweight-bearing exercises, such as water sports and activities, can be used if land-based weight-bearing exercises cause pain.

❖ Asthma-related deaths in the United States number more than 5,000 annually.

❖ The American Academy of Allergy and Immunology encourages asthmatics to exercise regularly.

❖ Exercise-induced asthma occurs from the loss of respiratory heat and water resulting from rapid breathing rates.

❖ Of the many forms of exercise, swimming and other water activities are the least asthmogenic.

❖ Clinical depression—prolonged sadness that persists beyond a reasonable time—responds to regular exercise.

Notes

1. S. L. Murphy, "Deaths: Final Data for 1998," *National Vital Statistics Report,* 48:11 (July 24, 2000).

2. American Heart Association, *1999 Heart and Stroke Statistical Update* (Dallas: AHA, 1998).

3. S. Margolis and G. Gerstenblith, *Coronary Heart Disease* (Baltimore: Johns Hopkins Medical Institution, 2001).

4. AHA, Note 2.

5. L. K. Smith, S. Brener, and F. J. Pashkow, "Medical and Invasive Interventions in the Management of Coronary Artery Disease," *ACSM's Resource Manual,* edited by J. L. Roitman (Philadelphia: Lippincott Williams and Wilkins, 2001).

6. AHA, Note 2.

7. H. B. Simon, *Preventing Heart Disease* (Palm Coast, FL: Harvard Health Publications, 2000).

8. Simon, Note 7.

9. "Old Habits: Will You Pay for Your Past as a Smoker?" *Harvard Health Letter,* 23:8 (June 1998), 1–3.

10. B. L. Marks, "Tobacco Exposure and Chronic Illness," *ACSM's Resource Manual*, edited by J. L. Roitman (Philadelphia: Lippincott Williams and Wilkins, 2001).

11. American Cancer Society, *Cancer Facts and Figures 2001* (Atlanta: ACS, 2001).

12. ACS, Note 11.

13. American College of Sports Medicine, "Physical Activity, Physical Fitness, and Hypertension," *Medicine and Science in Sports and Exercise*, 25:10 (1993), i.

14. J. Hagberg et al., "Exercise Training Helps Control Blood Pressure," *The Fit Society Page* (Winter, 1997), p. 5.

15. K. J. Stewart, "Exercise and Hypertension," *ACSM's Resource Manual*, edited by J. L. Roitman (Philadelphia: Lippincott Williams and Wilkins, 2001).

16. Stewart, Note 15.

17. "Revised Cholesterol Guidelines," *Harvard Heart Letter*, 11:11 (July 2001): 6–7.

18. J. C. La Rosa et al., "The Cholesterol Facts: A Summary of the Evidence Relating to Dietary Fats, Serum Cholesterol, and Coronary Heart Disease: A Joint Statement by the American Heart Association and the National Heart, Lung, and Blood Institute," *Circulation*, 81 (1990), 1721.

19. Simon, Note 7.

20. D. C. Nieman, *Exercise Testing and Prescription: A Health-Related Approach* (Mountain View, CA: Mayfield, 1999).

21. Simon, Note 7.

22. J. D. Potter and F. Hutchinson, "Hazards and Benefits of Alcohol," *New England Journal of Medicine*, 337:24 (Dec. 11, 1997), 1763–1764.

23. Simon, Note 7.

24. Margolis and Gerstenblith, Note 3.

25. I-M Lee, C. Hsieh, and R. S. Paffenbarger, "Exercise Intensity and Longevity in Men: The Harvard Alumni Health Study," *Journal of the American Medical Association*, 273:5 (April 19, 1995), 1179–1184.

26. S. N. Blair et al., "Changes in Physical Fitness and All-Cause Mortality," *Journal of the American Medical Association*, 273:14 (April 12, 1995), 1093–1098.

27. K. E. Powell et al., "Physical Activity and the Incidence of Coronary Heart Disease," *Annual Review of Public Health*, 8 (1987), 253.

28. M. A. Mittleman et al., "Triggering of Acute Myocardial Infarction by Heavy Physical Exertion," *New England Journal of Medicine*, 329 (1993), 1677.

29. S. N. Willich et al., "Physical Exertion as a Trigger of Acute Myocardial Infarction," *New England Journal of Medicine*, 329 (1993), 1684.

30. NHLBI, *Obesity Education Initiative Expert Panel Clinical Guidelines on the Identification, Evaluation and Treatment of Overweight and Obesity in Adults* (Washington, DC: National Heart, Lung, and Blood Institute, 1998).

31. ACS, Note 11.

32. Margolis and Gerstenblith, Note 3.

33. ACSM, *Guidelines for Exercise Testing and Prescription* (Philadelphia: Lippincott Williams and Wilkins, 2000).

34. D. Schardt, and S. Schmidt, "How to Avoid Adult Onset Diabetes," *Nutrition Action Healthletter*, 23:7 (Sept 1996), 3-5.

35. J. E. Manson et al., "A Prospective Study of Exercise and Incidence of Diabetes Among U. S. Male Physicians," *Journal of the American Medical Association*, 268 (1992), 268.

36. S. Poindexter, L. St. Clair, and K. Wheeler, "Diet and Chronic Disease," *ACSM's Resource Manual*, edited by J. L. Roitman (Philadelphia: Lippincott Williams and Wilkins, 2001).

37. Margolis and Gerstenblith, Note 3.

38. Margolis and Gerstenblith, Note 3.

39. ACS, Note 11.

40. ACS, Note 11.

41. Poindexter, St. Clair, and Wheeler, Note 36.

42. "Regular Physical Exertion May Fight Cancer as Well as Heart Disease," *Tufts University Health and Nutrition Letter*, 18:7 (Sept. 2000), 3.

43. I-M. Lee, "Exercise and Physical Health: Cancer and Immune Function," *Research Quarterly in Exercise and Sports*, 66 (1995), 86–291.

44. "The Quest for Healthy Bones" University of California at Berkeley *Wellness Letter*, 17:7 (April 2001), 4–5.

45. A. L. Fassler and J. P. Bonjour, "Osteoporosis as a Pediatric Problem," *Pediatrics Clinics of North America*, 42 (1995) 811–824.

46. F. D. Wolinsky, J. F. Fitzgerald, and T. E. Stump, "The Effect of Hip Fracture on Mortality, Hospitalization, and Functional Status: A Prospective Study," *American Journal of Public Health*, 87 (1997) 398–403.

47. J. M. Shaw, K. A. Witzke and K. M. Winters, "Exercise for Skeletal Health and Osteoporosis Prevention," *ACSM's Resource Manual*, edited by J. L. Roitman (Philadelphia: Lippincott Williams and Wilkins, 2001).

48. ACSM, "Position Stand: Osteoporosis and Exercise," *Medicine and Science in Sports and Exercise*, 27:4 (1995), i–vii.

49. Shaw, Witzke, and Winters, Note 47.

50. D. T. Felson, "Obesity and Knee Osteoarthritis: The Framingham Study," *Annals of Internal Medicine*, 109 (1988), 18.

51.   D. T. Felson, "Weight and Osteoarthritis," *American Journal of Clinical Nutrition*, 63 (Suppl) (1996), 4305–4325.

52. C. X. Bryant, J. A. Peterson, and J. E. Graves, "Muscular Strength and Endurance," *ACSM's Resource Manual,* edited by J. L. Roitman (Philadelphia: Lippincott Williams and Wilkins, 2001).

53. F. S. Sanders, "Exercise Induced Asthma in Athletes," *ACSM Certified News* 7:3 (Dec. 1997), 1–3.

54. C. C. W. Hsia, "Pathophysiology of Lung Disease," *ACSM's Resource Manual,* edited by J. L. Roitman (Philadelphia: Lippincott Williams and Wilkins, 2001).

55. Sanders, Note 53.

56. R. Scales and J. Blumenthal, "Influence of Emotional Distress on Chronic Illness," *ACSM's Resource Manual*, edited by J. L. Roitman (Philadelphia: Lippincott Williams and Wilkins, 2001).

57. Nieman, Note 20.

Appendix

World Wide Web Sites of Interest

ACSM's Health and Fitness Journal

www.health-fitjrnl.com/

> A journal published by Lippincott Williams and Wilkins for the American College of Sports Medicine, written for laypersons; covers a gamut of articles about exercise, sports, nutrition, injuries, and many more.

American Heart Association (AHA)

www.americanheart.org/

> National directory of resources related to heart health and disease.

American Institute for Cancer Research

www.aicr.org/

> Provides lifestyle recommendations for cancer prevention, as well as healthful recipes, research news, and links to cancer and nutrition resources.

American Running Association

www.americanrunning.org/

> A nonprofit educational association of runners, medical professionals, and corporations dedicated to promoting running nationwide; for more than 30 years the American Running Association and its sister organization, the American Medical Athletic Association, have been influential clearinghouses, providing information and support to runners nationwide.

American Running and Fitness Association

Key word on AOL is ARFA

> A collection of information and links related to running, swimming, cycling, nutrition, and other fitness activities.

Anorexia Nervosa and Related Eating Disorders

www.anred.com

> Provides information about anorexia nervosa, bulimia nervosa, binge eating disorder, compulsive exercising, and other less well-known food and weight disorders.

Centers for Disease Control and Prevention (CDC)

www.governmentguide.com

> Offered by the lead federal agency for protecting the health and safety of people at home and abroad, providing credible information to enhance health decisions and promoting health through strong partnerships.

Dr. Pribut's Running Injuries Page

www.drpribut.com/sports/sportframe.html

> Presented by a podiatrist, discussing common injures including achilles tendonitis, iliotibial band syndrome, runner's knee problems, ankle sprains, plantar fasciitis, shin splints, neuroma pain, hamstring injuries, and many others; provides tips on stretching, running in hot and cold weather, and other topics.

Food and Drug Administration (FDA)

www.governmentquide.com

> An agency that promotes public health by reviewing clinical research and taking appropriate action on the marketing of regulated products.

International Association of Fitness Professionals

www.ideafit.com

> Has a mission to support the world's leading health and fitness professionals with credible information on education, career-development, and leadership to help enhance the quality of life worldwide through participation in safe, effective fitness, and healthy lifestyle programs.

International Sports Sciences Association

www.fitnesscertification.com

>A fitness certification agency for personal trainers, strength coaches, aerobics instructors, and other exercise enthusiasts.

National Diabetes Information Clearinghouse

www.niddk.nih.gov

>Conducts and suggests basic and clinical research into diabetes, as well as digestive and kidney diseases.

National Institute on Aging

www.nih.gov/nia

>Has a mission to improve the health and well-being of older Americans through research and dissemination of pertinent information.

National Institute of Health (NIH)

www.nih.gov

>Dedicated to uncovering new knowledge that will lead to better health for everyone by conducting research, supporting research in universities, medical schools, and the like, by assisting in the training of research investigators, and fostering communication of medical information.

National Mental Health Association

www.mnha.org

>The oldest and largest nonprofit organization in the United States addressing all aspects of mental health and mental illness.

National Osteoporosis Foundation

www.nof.org

>Provides information on the causes, prevention, detection, and treatment of osteoporosis, including risk factors and general bone health.

National Strength and Conditioning Association

www.nsca-lift.org

>An organization of exercise and medical science specialists whose common interest is strength conditioning for athletic performance.

North American Association for the Study of Obesity

www.maaso.org/

>An interdisciplinary society whose purpose is to develop, extend, and disseminate knowledge in the field of obesity.

Physician and Sportsmedicine

www.physsportsmed.com/

>A journal covering practical, primary-care oriented topics such as diagnosing and treating knee and ankle injuries, managing chronic disease, preventing and managing overuse injuries, helping people lose weight safely, and the range of exercise and nutrition topics.

President's Council on Physical Fitness and Sports

www.fitness.gov

>Serves as a catalyst to promote, encourage, and motivate Americans of all ages to become physically active and participate in sports; advises the U.S. President and Secretary of Health and Human Services on how to encourage more Americans to be physically fit and active.

Runner's World

www.runnersworld.com/

>Informs, advises, educates, and motivates runners of all ages and abilities: "We want to help every runner achieve his/her personal health, fitness, and performance goals."

Sports, Cardiovascular, and Wellness Nutritionists

www.nutrifit.org

>An organization that pursues professional excellence in sports and cardiovascular nutrition, wellness, and disordered eating by providing professional development and networking opportunities to members.

U.S. Department of Health and Human Services

www.os.dhhs.gov

>The U.S. government's principal agency for protecting the health of all Americans and providing essential human services, especially for those who are least able to help themselves; offers more than 300 programs covering a wide spectrum of activities.

Glossary

Adipose tissue Fat cells in the body.

Aerobic Literally meaning "with oxygen."

Aerobic capacity Maximal amount of oxygen the human body is able to utilize per minute of physical activity (usually expressed in ml/kg/min).

Aerobic exercise Activity that requires oxygen to produce the necessary energy to carry out the activity.

Allergen Any substance that produces an allergic response.

Amino acids Chemical compounds that contain nitrogen, carbon, hydrogen, and oxygen; basic building blocks the body uses to build different types of protein.

Amenorrhea Cessation of the menstrual cycle.

Anabolism The assimilation of nutrients and their conversion to living tissue.

Anaerobic Literally meaning "without oxygen."

Anaerobic exercise High-intensity activity that does not require oxygen to produce the desired energy.

Anaerobic threshold The point during exercise at which blood lactate suddenly begins to increase.

Android obesity Masculine pattern of body fat deposition in the abdomen, chest, and back.

Antioxidant Compounds such as vitamins C, E, beta-carotene, and selenium that prevent oxygen from combining with other substances it may damage.

Arterioles Smallest arteries in the body.

Asthmogenic Substances or events that are capable of producing bronchospasms.

Atherosclerosis A slow, progressive disease of large and medium-size arteries characterized by the formation of plaque; implicated in heart disease. Responsible for 80% of coronary artery disease.

Atrophy Decrease or shrinkage in the size of a cell caused by disuse for whatever reason.

Ballistic stretching Exercises done using jerky, rapid, and bouncy movements.

Basal metabolic rate (BMR) Minimum amount of energy the body expends to sustain life while at complete rest.

Blood plasma Liquid portion of the blood.

Body composition Proportionate amounts of fat and lean body tissues.

Body mass index (BMI) Ratio of weight to height; used to determine thinness and fatness and risk for disease.

Carcinogenic Describes substances that are capable of producing cancer.

Cardiac output (Q) Represents the amount of blood pumped by the heart in 1 minute.

Cardiac reserve The difference between HR max and RHR.

Cardiorespiratory endurance Ability of the lungs, heart, and blood vessels to deliver adequate amounts of oxygen to the cells to meet the demands of prolonged physical activity.

Cardiovascular disease Any illness of the heart and coronary blood vessels.

Catabolism Breakdown of complex chemical compounds into simpler ones for use by the body.

Catecholamines The hormones epinephrine and norepinephrine; stimulants to the circulatory system that constrict blood vessels.

Chronic diseases Longlasting and/or frequently occurring illnesses.

Chronic stress Long-term stress induced by persistent exposure to a stressor or group of stressors.

Clinical depression Prolonged sadness that persists for some time without an identified cause (in contrast to situational depression).

Communicable Describes diseases that can be transmitted from outside agents; also called infectious diseases.

Concentric muscle contraction A reaction in which the muscle shortens while the individual lifts a weight against the force of gravity.

Conduction Heat loss by physical contact between two objects.

Convection Heat loss that occurs when a cooler gas or liquid flows across the skin.

Cool-Down A period of time following exercise consisting of mild activity that prevents the pooling of blood in the leg veins. This technique allows the body to safely return to the rested state.

Coronary heart disease (CHD) Illness of the heart caused by atherosclerotic narrowing of the coronary arteries.

Cross-training Exercise format that utilizes a variety of activities rather than just one.

Cryotherapy Use of cold applications in the treatment of injuries.

Dehydration Excessive loss of fluid from the body.

Degenerative disease Chronic illness that becomes progressively worse over time.

Delayed onset muscle soreness Soreness that usually occurs 24 to 48 hours after a vigorous workout in which eccentric muscle contractions have taken place.

Depression Prolonged sadness that persists beyond a reasonable time.

Diastolic blood pressure The pressure between heartbeats when the heart is at rest and filling with blood.

Disuse atrophy Premature loss resulting from understimulation.

Diuretic Refers to substances that cause the body to excrete excess water through urine.

DNA Master blueprint for cellular function.

Duration How long a person exercises.

Dynamic stretching Stretching that involves bouncing and bobbing movements.

Eccentric muscle contraction Lengthening a muscle while resisting the force of gravity as it returns to the starting position.

Edema Swelling of a body part that results from accumulation of fluid.

Electrocardiograph (ECG) Measurement of electric activity of the heart.

Electrolytes Ions that conduct electricity.

Essential fat Body fat that is indispensable to normal physiological functioning.

Essential hypertension Persistent high blood pressure that has no known cause.

Estrogen Steroid hormone secreted primarily by the ovaries; involved in the development and maintenance of female reproductive organs, secondary sexual characteristics, and the menstrual cycle.

Evaporation Loss of body heat when liquid sweat is vaporized at surface of the skin.

Exercise electrocardiogram (ECG) An exercise test during which the workload is gradually increased (until the subject reaches maximal fatigue) with blood pressure and 12-lead electrocardiographic monitoring throughout the test.

Exercise heart rate The heart rate that an exerciser needs to maintain to improve aerobic capacity.

Epinephrine Hormone secreted by the adrenal glands that constricts blood vessels.

Estrogen Female sex hormone thought to contribute to some disease conditions.

External (extrinsic) rewards Reinforcement administered by outside sources.

Flexibility Range of movement around joints of the body.

Folic acid B vitamin necessary for controlling blood level of homocysteine.

Free radicals Byproducts of oxidation that damage cells and DNA.

Frequency Number of times per week a person participates in physical activity.

Goal An end or objective to be achieved.

Gynoid obesity The feminine pattern of body fat deposition in the hips, buttocks, and thighs.

HDL High density lipoproteins, which scavenge cholesterol from tissues and bloodstream and transfer it back to the liver through intermediary carriers, for degradation, recycling, or disposal; "good cholesterol."

Health promotion Fostering lifestyle behaviors that enhance health, such as exercise, smoking cessation, blood pressure screening, cholesterol evaluation, stress management, and weight control.

Health-related fitness Fitness goal that emphasizes development of cardiorespiratory endurance, muscular strength and endurance, flexibility, and lean body composition.

Heart rate reserve (HRR) Difference between maximal heart rate and resting heart rate.

Heat exhaustion A reaction to heat, marked by prostration, weakness, and collapse resulting from severe dehydration.

Heat stroke A severe and often fatal illness produced by exposure to excessively high temperatures, especially when accompanied by vigorous physical exertion.

Hematocrit Ratio of red blood cells to plasma volume.

Hemoglobin Iron pigment of red blood cells that carries oxygen and carbon dioxide.

Homeostasis State of equilibrium with respect to body functions and to the chemical composition of fluids and tissues.

Homocysteine One of the amino-acid building blocks of protein; high levels damage arteries.

Hormone replacement therapy (HRT) Replacing estrogen in the female, usually after menopause, when its natural production stops.

Hydrogenated Describes the process whereby hydrogen is added to fats to increase shelf life and make the product more spreadable; increases saturation of the fat.

Hypertension Medical term for high blood pressure

Hyperthermia Excessive heat accumulation in the body.

Hypothermia Excessive heat lost from the body.

Inflammation Disease condition produced by infection, injury, or irritant, characterized by redness, swelling, and pain.

Insoluble fiber Dietary fiber in polysaccharides that is insoluble in hot water; enhances the health of the intestines by speeding food remnants through them.

Insulin Hormone manufactured by the body that facilitates passage of sugar from blood to cells.

Intensity Amount of energy expended per bout of exercise.

Internal (intrinsic) rewards Reinforcement coming from within; no visible reward.

Interval training A type of intermittent training featuring cycles of very high-intensity, short-duration activities followed by short periods of active rest, such as walking.

Ischemia Diminished blood flow to the heart.

Karvonen method One of the more accurate methods of determining exercise heart rate. This method uses the cardiac reserve and the individual's physical fitness level to calculate the training heart rate.

Kilocalories (kcals) Measurement of the number of calories found in food; also called calories.

Lactate threshold The point during exercise at which blood lactate suddenly begins to increase. Accumulation of lactate interferes with muscle contraction and is detrimental to performance.

LDL Low density lipoproteins, which transport cholesterol from liver to body cells; "bad cholesterol."

Lipids Scientific term for fats in the blood.

Lipoproteins Carriers to which cholesterol attaches for transport through the circulatory system.

Lp(a) Lipoprotein (a), which in high levels can promote development of blood clots in the arteries.

Macronutrients One of two categories of minerals also known as major minerals; the other category is micronutrients.

Malignant Describes tumors or tissues that are cancerous.

Maximal heart rate (MHR) Highest heart rate for a person, primarily related to age.

Menopause Decline and eventual cessation of hormone production by reproductive system in midlife; termination of menstrual cycle.

Menstruation Monthly flow of blood from uterine lining; also termed *menses*.

Metabolic diseases Category of diseases involving body metabolism, including diabetes mellitus, thyroid disorders, kidney disease, and liver disease.

Metabolic syndrome Characterized by abdominal obesity, insulin resistance, high LDLs, high triglycerides, high blood pressure, and low HDLs.

Metabolism Sum of chemical changes occurring in tissues, consisting of anabolism and catabolism.

Metastasis Spread of cancer from its original site to other areas of the body.

Micronutrients Trace minerals; nutrients in quantities less than 5 grams.

Monounsaturated fatty acid A healthier form of fat characterized by one carbon-to-carbon double bond.

Morbidity Sick rate in a population.

Mortality Death rate in a population.

Motivation Internal mechanisms and external stimuli that arouse and stimulate behavior.

Muscular endurance Capacity to exert repetitive muscular force.

Muscular strength Maximum amount of force that a muscle or group of muscles can exert in a single contraction.

Myocardial infarction Heart attack.

Myotatic reflex Response to forceful strength by a proprioceptor in the center of muscles.

Neoplasm New tissue or tumor.

Norepinephrine Hormone secreted by the adrenal glands that constricts blood vessels.

Nutrient density Ratio of nutrients to calories in food.

Nutrients Substances found in food that provide energy, regulate metabolism, and help with growth and repair of body tissues.

Obesity Chronic disease characterized by excessive body fat in relation to lean body mass.

Oncogene A cancerous gene.

Orthotics Orthopedic devices placed in shoes to correct biomechanical problems.

Osteoporosis Loss of bone mineral density that becomes apparent most often in postmenopausal women and elderly men.

Overfat Excessive fat: For males 23% to 25% or more of body weight is fat, and for females, 32% or more of body weight is fat.

Overload Subjecting the various body systems to greater physical demand to produce muscle development.

Overtraining The onset of physiological and psychological staleness brought about by exclusive exercise.

Overweight Excessive body weight for height.

Oxidation The process that transforms food materials into heat or mechanical energy.

Oxygen debt Amount of O_2 required during recovery from exercise that is over and above that which is normally required at rest.

Oxygen deficit The first 1 or 2 minutes of exercise when the O_2 demand exceeds the body's ability to supply it.

Oxygen drift A slight increase in oxygen consumption as a result of prolonged aerobic exercise.

Percent body fat Total amount of fat in the body based on the person's weight; includes both essential and storage fat.

Percent daily value Percentage of a food substance required daily..

Performance-related fitness Type of fitness that enables a person to perform physical skills with a high level of proficiency.

Peripheral vascular resistance Body condition in which the arterioles are in a constant state of slight contraction.

Peristalsis Waves of alternate contraction and relaxation that propel digested food along the colon.

Physical activity Bodily movement produced by skeletal muscles that requires energy expenditure and produces progressive health benefits.

Phytochemicals Compounds found in fruits and vegetables that block the formation of cancerous tumors and disrupt the process.

Phytoestrogens Plant estrogens that may protect against breast cancer.

Phytomedicinals Plants that have medicinal qualities.

Polyunsaturated fatty acids A healthier form of fat characterized by two or more carbon-to-carbon double bonds.

Positive feedback reinforcement A reward or action that increases the strength of a response.

Progression Exposing the body to greater and greater physical demands over time.

Proprioceptive neuromuscular facilitation (PNF) Stretching technique in which muscles are stretched progressively with intermittent isometric contractions.

Radiation Loss of body heat through electromagnetic waves emitted to the environment.

Rate of perceived exertion (RPE) A perception scale to monitor or interpret the intensity of aerobic exercise.

Recommended dietary allowance (RDA) Daily suggested intakes of nutrients for normal, healthy people, as developed by National Academy of Sciences.

Resting heart rate (RHR) Rate after a person has been sitting quietly for 15–20 minutes.

Resting metabolic rate (RMR) Amount of energy needed to sustain life in rested but awake state.

RICES An acronym that stands for rest, ice, compression, elevation, and stabilization of an injured body part.

Risk factors Genetic tendencies and learned behaviors that increase the probability of premature illness and death from specific diseases.

Self-motivation Desire to persist at a task without constant help or praise.

Serum cholesterol Cholesterol level in the blood.

Skinfold thickness Technique to assess body composition, including percent body fat, by measuring thickness of skin at specified body sites.

Soluble fiber Dietary fiber that dissolves in hot water.

Specificity of training A principle stating that training must be done with the specific muscle the body is attempting to improve.

Static stretching Holding muscle positions in a fixed manner for 15 to 30 seconds.

Storage fat Body fat in excess of the essential fat; stored in adipose tissue.

Stressors Any condition, circumstance, or event that provokes the stress response.

Stroke volume Amount of blood the heart can eject in one beat.

Systolic blood pressure Represents the pressure of the blood against the artery walls when the heart contracts.

Target heart rate Heart rate that should be attained during aerobic exercise that will result in improvement of aerobic capacity.

Thrombus Blood clot.

Transfatty acids Solidified fat formed by adding hydrogen to monosaturated and polyunsaturated fats to increase shelf life.

Triglycerides Fats formed by glycerol and three fatty acids.

Transtheoretical model for behavior change Behavioral theory characterized by stages of change.

Vasoconstriction Narrowing or clamping down of blood vessels.

Ventilation Amount of air moved in and out of the lungs in 1 minute.

VO$_2$ max Represents the body's peak ability to assimilate, deliver, and extract oxygen; considered to be the best indicator of physical fitness.

Weight cycling Repeated weight loss and regain; also called yo-yo dieting.

Waist/hip ratio A test to assess potential risk for diseases based on body fat pattern distribution.

Warm-up A period of time prior to exercise that prepares the body for physical activity by slowly increasing heart rate and muscle temperature.

Index